VETERINARY SCIENCES AND MEDICINE

ANTHELMINTICS

CLINICAL PHARMACOLOGY, USES IN VETERINARY MEDICINE AND EFFICACY

VETERINARY SCIENCES AND MEDICINE

Additional books in this series can be found on Nova's website under the Series tab.

Additional e-books in this series can be found on Nova's website under the e-book tab.

VETERINARY SCIENCES AND MEDICINE

ANTHELMINTICS

CLINICAL PHARMACOLOGY, USES IN VETERINARY MEDICINE AND EFFICACY

WILLIAM QUICK
EDITOR

NOVA BIOMEDICAL

New York

For permission to use material from this book please contact us:
Telephone 631-231-7269; Fax 631-231-8175
Web Site: http://www.novapublishers.com

Library of Congress Cataloging-in-Publication Data

ISBN: 978-1-63117-714-9
LCCN: 2014936327

Published by Nova Science Publishers, Inc. † New York

Contents

Preface

Antiparasitic drugs (ATH) are important tools widely used to maintain animal welfare. As parasites impart a great impact on animal health, these drugs are often essential for the expression of the full genetic potential of production. However, despite the initial success, after years of massive use of anthelminthic drugs, the increase in prevalence of resistant nematodes became a major problem. Anthelmintics are commonly used to treat parasitic worm infections not only in animals, but humans as well. Resistance to anthelmintics is thought to be present in several helminth species, yet it remains poorly studied. This book discusses topics such as the clinical pharmacology of anthelmintics; the uses in human and veterinary medicine; animal resistance to ATH; and the efficacy of Neem and Pawpaw products against Oesophahostomum spp infection in pigs.

Chapter 1 - The efficacy of phenotypic assessments to detect anthelmintic resistance can fluctuate substantially. In some cases, the level of anthel-mintic resistance may be overestimated. The main factors associated with "false resistance" include: the use of low quality drugs (some generic drugs), poor absorption or metabolisation of the drug, or, under dosing. Conversely, anthelmintic resistance may be underestimated due to lack of reliable indicators and surveys. Anthelmintic resistance has been almost entirely studied in gastro-intestinal nematodes (GIN), although resistance has also been demonstrated or suspected in liver fluke and the cestode Moniezia. Determining anthelmintic resistance in GIN field studies is based exclusively on phenotypic evaluation, the evolution of faecal egg counts before and after a treatment, and in a few instances, on actual worm counts.

Several important points need to be considered in determining the reliability of GIN faecal egg counts such as: i) the sampling procedure of faeces (individual or composite), ii) the sampled animals (high versus low infection level, number of samples) iii) the moment of sampling after treatment (long enough to detect a decrease in egg counts but not too long so reinfection could then interfere with results), and iv) the mode of calculation (based on individual or average efficacy, each of which has several potential methods of calculation). In this chapter, the authors evaluate the relative importance of each of these four points. To do this, they gather results from various studies obtained from the literature and from as yet unpublished original research from their own datasets and from those provided by other researchers. The authors conclude by discussing the potential of using faecal egg counts as an indicator to evaluate anthelmintic resistance, and its place in GIN management.

Chapter 2 - Anthelmintics are commonly used to treat parasitic worm infections in human and animals. These parasitic worms infect crops, domestic pets and livestock. Helminth, being tropical infectious disease gets less attention from developed world. The main chemotherapeutic agents used in humans are mainly adapted from veterinary medicine. Among them only few drugs have a broad spectrum activity while many drugs have very limited action against particular species. The few parameters like dosing frequency of anthelmintics, efficacy of drug, degree of infection and untreated population of parasitic worms in body affects the possibility of deve-lopping resistance both in human and animals.

However, various academics institutes and industry are working on new ways and the types of drug delivery systems for anthelmintic drugs. In this chapter, the current chemotherapy in veterinary and human medicine is reviewed. A detailed discussion on new drugs, formulation systems and clinical trial status is done at the end of chapter. The role of herbal antihelmintics is also discussed in detail. Special focus on the efficacy of various anthelmintic drugs in animals and human is given and debated.

Chapter 3 - *Trichostrongylid* nematodes are important parasites of domestic ruminants and are responsible for significant economic losses in tropical and temperate regions. After years of widespread use of anthelminthic drugs, the increasing prevalence of resistant nematodes now threatens the production of livestock in several parts of the world.

The continued drug use did not eradicate the parasites, mainly because the majority of the nematode populations are in *refugia* (e.g., eggs and larvae in the pasture or inside untreated asymptomatic animals), therefore not submitted to drug selection. Consequently, the genetic pool present in the populations in *refugia* continuously supply genetic variability, sometimes in the form of drug resistance conferring mutations, which eventually became fixed. The situation is further complicated by the high gene flow among parasite populations and their high mutation rates.

Indeed there are several reports describing that resistance can originate through different ways such as animal movement among farms and novel/recurrent mutations. Therefore considerable efforts are being made to develop tests for the diagnosis of anthelminthic resistance that would allow the establishment of rational and sustainable programs for the control of nematode populations in livestock. In this context, molecular tests based on the analysis of resistance-associated target gene polymorphisms become attractive since they present high sensitivity and can deliver precise results in shorter periods of time than traditional techniques.

A major drawback for the development of molecular tests, though, is the poor knowledge about the genetic mutations associated with the resistant phenotypes for most drug classes. In here, it is described the current knowledge about the molecular basis of anthelminthic drug resistance and the prevalence of resistance in different *Trichostrongylid* species. Anthelminthic drug resistance rise and spread is also discussed in the context of nematode population genetics dynamics.

Chapter 4 - The gastrointestinal helminthes are major limiting factors for the sheep and goat production in the world and the health of livestock depends of effective control of nematodes. The constant administration and inadequate doses of chemical anthelmintics favors the selection of resistant populations and residues these products contribute to the contamination of animal products and of the ambient. The use of herbal treatment in veterinary medicine is a promising field of research. Studies in this area require the insertion into an agroecological context, with the limiting factor to the sustainable management of natural resources involved. The phytotherapy for the parasite control is an alternative that can reduce the cost with the purchase of anthelmintics as well, preventing the emergence of anthelmintic resistance and residues in animal products. Plant species that have tannins in its constitution are known to possess anthelmintic activity, requiring, however, that their efficacies are scientifically proven. The Cerrado is an import biome with high diversity of plants rich in tannins and other metabolic with potential anthelmintic effect. This study presents a review of research on plant species, tested in the Cerrado for the control of helminths in ruminants.

Chapter 5 - Millions of humans and animals are simultaneously infected with different helminth species. However, an important group of disease-causing organisms has often been excluded from such surveys, namely the zoonotic larval cestodoses. In 2007, the World Health Organization included echinococcosis and cysticercosis as a part of a neglected zoonosis subgroup for its strategic plan for the control of neglected tropical diseases (NTDs). Praziquantel (PZQ) has a remarkable range of activity that has been shown to be effective against cestodes and trematodes. It is considered as a drug of choice to control all forms of schistosomiasis in humans and animals. Although it is very well tolerated, and has relatively low level of toxicity and few side effects, much remains to be learned about drug disposition. The very high cost of discovering and developing of new drugs is reflected in the limited number of new classes of antiparasitic agents launched on the market. To identify the new antiparasitic lead compounds, very many compounds will have to be examined in pre-clinical tests. Therefore there is the need of alternative treatment approaches. PZQ has limited water-solubility in biofluids, the result of which is that only a low concentration of the active drug can reach parasites localized in the parenchymal tissues. In this respect, modified drug formulations, which could overcome this problem, can lead to the improvement of efficacy. Spherical lipid vesicles such are liposomes are made from natural lipids and offer many advantages as drug carriers. Immunosuppression of host immune responses, triggered by parasite-derived molecules, is a phenomenon characteristic of helminth infections, and can be manipulated with some drugs (e.g., PZQ) and especially with external immunomodulatory substances. Until a new compound with antiparasitic effect and simultaneous stimulatory activity towards the host´s immunity is available, safe and cheap alternative approaches need to be investigated. There are a numerous compounds isolated from natural sources without having toxic side-effects, which are currently evaluated in antiparasitic therapy, either as single drugs or in combination with current drugs. *Mesocestoides vogae* (syn. *Mesocestoides corti*, Etges, 1991) is considered as a good experimental model to study cestode biology and the effects of drugs, because it can be easily manipulated both *in vivo* and *in vitro* and due to its relatively close relationship with cestodes of medical relevance, such as species of *Echinococcus* or *Taenia*.

The findings summarised in this chapter demonstrate that the efficacy of praziquantel towards larval cestodes can be markedly improved after their incorporation into suitable liposomal drug carriers and application of the immunomodulatory substances, glucan and silymarin offered a very effective tool to activate cells of host immune defence system, which is immunosuppressed towards Th2 response. Finally, the authors' therapeutical approach to combine drugs entrapped in carriers with liposomized glucan or silymarin proved to have multiple advantages over the classical therapy, regarding the efficacy and host pathophysiology.

Chapter 6 - Plant based remedies are used by pig farmers in control of nematode parasites, although their efficacies has not been evaluated under *in-vitro* and *in-vivo* experiments. Pawpaw and neem products are commonly used as anthelmintics by farmers in Kenya to control of livestock nematodes. The current study evaluated the efficacy of these products using *in-vitro* and *in-vivo* methods. In the first study, the efficacies of pawpaw and neem products against various stages of *Oesophagostomum* spp were tested under laboratory conditions. The *Oesophagostomum* spp eggs from pigs were exposed to various concentrations of pawpaw, neem products and commercial papain using *in vitro* assays.

Papain and pawpaw latex were the most effective products against *Oesophagostomum* spp, the most lethal effect being on egg hatching with an ED50 ranging between 5 and 59 μg/ml. The adult worms' ED50 was 12.5μg/ml for papain and 25μg/ml for pawpaw latex. In adult worms, the paw paw latex caused the cuticle to disintegrate leading to exposure of internal organs. 100% mortality was observed in adult worms exposed to neem oil concentrations of 25% or higher. The *in vitro* study showed that pawpaw and neem extracts have significant anthelmintics potential. In the second *in vivo* study, the efficacies of pawpaw and neem products were investigated in pigs. Thirty (30) pigs with natural infection of *Oesophago-stomum* spp were treated orally with pawpaw latex (1g/Kg), pawpaw seeds powder (1g/Kg), papain (0.3g/Kg), neem oil (0.2ml/Kg) and levamisole (7.5mg/kg) and monitored for egg counts for 56 days post treatment (dpt). Six pigs were also kept as untreated controls. Fecal samples were collected weekly from the pigs and analysed for eggs per gram (EPG) using the McMaster method. Other parameters which were monitored included clinical signs, packed cell volume (PCV) of collected blood and weight changes. The study showed a decline in EPG counts of pigs treated with all the products, with the percentage reductions in EPG at 56dpt in the levamisole, latex, neem, papain, powder treated pigs at 84.6%, 57.1%, 56%, 43.2%, 27.1%, respectively. A rise in mean EPGs (47% at 56 dpt) was observed in the untreated control groups. Significant differences ($p<0.05$) were observed between mean EPGs in the following groups: untreated controls and latex, levamisole and neem groups. There were no clinical signs observed in the treated pigs and the weight gain ranged from 111g to 145g/pig/day, but the weight differences amongst the various groups were not ($p>0.05$) significant. There was an increase in PCV in pigs from all the treatment groups which was higher than that of the untreated control group. It is concluded that, pawpaw products and neem oil used at the current dosages were safe and significant effect against *Oesophagostomum* spp infection in pigs. Further studies on the pawpaw and neem oil products including dosage formulation and effectiveness of the products in integrated control programmes for pig parasites are recommended.

In: Anthelmintics
Editor: William Quick
ISBN: 978-1-63117-714-9

Chapter 1

Reliable Phenotypic Evaluations of Anthelmintic Resistance in Herbivores: How and When Should They Be Done?

J. Cabaret[*]
INRA and F. Rabelais University Tours, Nouzilly, France

Abstract

The efficacy of phenotypic assessments to detect anthelmintic resistance can fluctuate substantially. In some cases, the level of anthelmintic resistance may be overestimated. The main factors associated with "false resistance" include: the use of low quality drugs (some generic drugs), poor absorption or metabolisation of the drug, or, under dosing. Conversely, anthelmintic resistance may be underestimated due to lack of reliable indicators and surveys. Anthelmintic resistance has been almost entirely studied in gastro-intestinal nematodes (GIN), although resistance has also been demonstrated or suspected in liver fluke and the cestode Moniezia. Determining anthelmintic resistance in GIN field studies is based exclusively on phenotypic evaluation, the evolution of faecal egg

[*] Corresponding author: J. Cabaret. INRA and F. Rabelais University Tours, UMR 1282, 37380 Nouzilly, France. E-mail: cabaret@tours.inra.fr.

counts before and after a treatment, and in a few instances, on actual worm counts.

Several important points need to be considered in determining the reliability of GIN faecal egg counts such as: i) the sampling procedure of faeces (individual or composite), ii) the sampled animals (high versus low infection level, number of samples) iii) the moment of sampling after treatment (long enough to detect a decrease in egg counts but not too long so reinfection could then interfere with results), and iv) the mode of calculation (based on individual or average efficacy, each of which has several potential methods of calculation). In this chapter, we evaluate the relative importance of each of these four points. To do this, we gather results from various studies obtained from the literature and from as yet unpublished original research from our own datasets and from those provided by other researchers. We conclude by discussing the potential of using faecal egg counts as an indicator to evaluate anthelmintic resistance, and its place in GIN management.

Introduction

Resistance to anthelmintics is thought to be present in several helminth species, yet it remains poorly studied. For example, while resistance to triclabendazole has been recorded in liver fluke (Mooney et al., 2009 and Oleachea et al. 2011) few studies are available which document the extent of its prevalence. The majority of what we know in this area is based on studies with gastro-intestinal nematodes (GIN) and as such, we will concentrate on them specifically within this chapter. Anthelmintic resistance in GIN is widespread in farmed ruminants and it continues to increase (Overend et al., 1994; van Wyk et al., 1998; Kaplan 2004; Cabaret and Silvestre, 2012).

Its prevalence is variable from one host species to another with goats (mostly dairy goats from developed countries) considered to be the most likely to harbor anthelmintic resistant worm populations, whereas cattle are the least likely (Demeler et al., 2009). The increase of anthelmintic resistance in GIN is particularly important in horses with the index rising from 6% (records from 1973-1999) to 34% (1973 - 2011). During this period, the increase was found to be less important in goats (30 to 43%) or sheep (22 to 35%) and relatively unchanged in cattle (17 to 15%) (Cabaret and Silvestre, 2012). Anthelmintic resistance occurs in nearly all species of GIN, with the *Haemonchus* species found to be the most commonly resistant species to benzimidazoles.

Several factors exist which may lead to false indications of anthelmintic resistance in GIN including: low quality drugs (some generic drugs), the use of drugs exceeding their shelf-life, poor absorption or metabolisation of the drug, a particularly important issue in goat treatment (Cabaret, 2010), under-dosing due to incorrect estimates of ruminant live-weight, an important determinant in deciding upon adequate dose levels, or using the incorrect drug to treat specific GIN species (for example Closantel use should be restricted to blood sucking parasites). With the exception of benzimidazoles, we lack resistance diagnostics pertaining to the varying modes of action of the anthelmintics. As a result, we rely almost exclusively on the use of phenotypic tests to evaluate anthelmintic resistance. The methods of such tests are a potential source for under or over-estimation of GIN anthelmintic resistance in themselves.

This chapter will firstly present the main anthelmintics used against GIN, their respective modes of action and the appearance of resistance against them, and the tests available to detect anthelmintic resistance. We will then study in greater detail the most commonly used test, e.g., the faecal egg count reduction test. Finally, we conclude by discussing the means for optimal detection of anthelmintic resistance in order to choose the most adequate anthelmintic(s) in the control of GIN.

I. The Main Anthelmintics and the Appearance of Resistance

a) Their Modes of Action and Consequence for Resistance (Table 1)

There are 11 different modes of actions for anthelmintics (Robertson et al., 2012) and six related to GIN are recorded in table 1.

There is no cross resistance between anthelmintics with different modes of action. Within a group of anthelmintics sharing the same mode of action, the resistance to one drug is also expected to be present against the other drugs in the group. This is perfectly true for the anthelmintics acting on the tubulin ligands activity: the GIN are resistant to all the benzimidazoles. This is less true for macrocyclic lactones and for cholinergic agonists (Charvet et al., 2012). The cholinergic anthelmintics, pyrantel and derquantel may still be effective on levamisole-resistant worms, another cholinergic anthelmintic, although it belongs in theory to the same cholinergic group. The structure of the different nicotinic receptors involved in resistance may explain these subtle resistance capacities among worms (Buxton et al., 2014). These results still need to be evidenced *in vivo* but the premise likely carries implications regarding how we manage drugs in anthelmintic resistant GIN.

Table 1. The main anthelmintics used in herbivores and the time taken for resistance to appear

Activity	Molecule	Year commercialised / number of years before resistance was first detected
Cholinergic agonist	Levamisole Pyrantel Monepantel	1970 / 9 1974 / 22 2010/ 3
Cholinergic antagonist	Derquantel (not available as a stand-alone drug)	2010
Glutamate Cl and GABA allosteric modulators	Ivermectin and other macrocyclic lactones.	1981 / 7
Calcium activated K channel activator	Emodepsine	Not used in herbivores although efficient
Tubulin ligands	Thiabendazole, and other benzimidazoles or a pro-benzimidazole (Netobimin)	1961 / 3
Oxydative phosphorylation/chitinase inhibitor	Closantel	1977/ 18

Modified from Cabaret and Silvestre 2012.

b) Time between Marketing of Anthelmintics and Appearance of GIN Resistance

The on-set of resistance varied in time for each specific anthelmintic, ranging from 3 years for thiabendazole and monepantel (Scott et al., 2013) to 18 years for closantel, with a maximum of 22 years for pyrantel.

While different breeding management factors (i.e., pasture type and use, the uncontrolled introduction of new hosts infected with resistant worms etc.) will play a role in the development of resistance to anthelmintics, it is likely these differences are predominantly a result of their differing resistance mechanisms.

For example, monogenic or nearly monogenic resistances such as for thiabendazole are more easily selected for than presumed polygenic ones such as levamisole or pyrantel.

The frequent use of the same treatment will also increase the selection rate of resistance (Barnes et al. 1995, Silvestre et al. 2002) the only unknown is at which speed it will occur.

This implies that monitoring resistance is an important task for the future control of GIN.

II. The Methods for Detecting Resistance: An Overview

The detection of anthelmintic resistance in GIN of veterinary importance has been reviewed on several occasions for each of the different species by the World Association for the Advancement of Veterinary Parasitology (WAAVP). The experimental efficacy of the anthelmintics has been based on worm counts in treated and untreated control animals following necropsy (for detailed examples see Duncan et al., 2002 in horses).

Determining the initial efficacy of an anthelmintic can be evaluated under strict experimental conditions using necropsies, and then the product, if efficient, may be distributed for use in farms.

There is therefore a need for accurate (species-specific when feasible), non-invasive techniques for evaluating anthelmintic resistance in living animals in farm conditions, which could be supported with worm counts at necropsy to a very limited extent.

Non-invasive techniques to count the GIN eggs or infective larvae are available but lack sensivity. Coles et al. (2006) reviewed these techniques as they apply to the main anthelmintics in all herbivore host species:

- Faecal egg count reduction test (FECRT): all drugs, all host species
- Egg hatch assay (EHA), valid for anthelmintics acting on egg hatching such as benzimidazoles, discriminating doses (eggs resistant versus susceptible GIN) only for sheep, goats and horses.
- Microagar larval development test: benzimidazole and levamisole in sheep, goats and horses where faecal egg counts are on average over 350 (preferably 500) eggs per gram in order to obtain enough larvae for statistical tests.

- Molecular tests based on PCR to detect resistance alleles: benzimidazoles, all host species

It is difficult to strictly compare these methods since they are not available for all the anthelmintics and such a comparison could only be made with reference to benzimidazoles (Figure 1). The greatest association between the estimates of these methods were found between molecular typing, EHA and worm counts in sheep GIN. While the EHA was related to molecular typing (Elard et al., 1999; Cudekova et al., 2010) this was only found to be true when 15% or more of the worm population was anthelmintic resistant. Bentounsi et al. (2007) found a significant correlation between EHA and FECRT in natural GIN infections with a similar coefficient of explanation- the square of correlation coefficient (48%) to experimental infections (40%) shown in Figure 1. Barrière et al. 2013 found a relationship between larval development test (12/13 farms detected as resistant to benzimidazoles) and FECRT (11/11 farms detected as resistant). The FECRT is able to detect resistance when more than 25% of the worms are resistant (Martin et al., 1989).

Although the poor sensitivity of the phenotypic methods were assessed relative only to benzimidazoles, there is no reason to expect that better results might be obtained for other drugs. These methods are able to detect resistance only when 20% of the worms are resistant: it means that we may detect already established resistances.

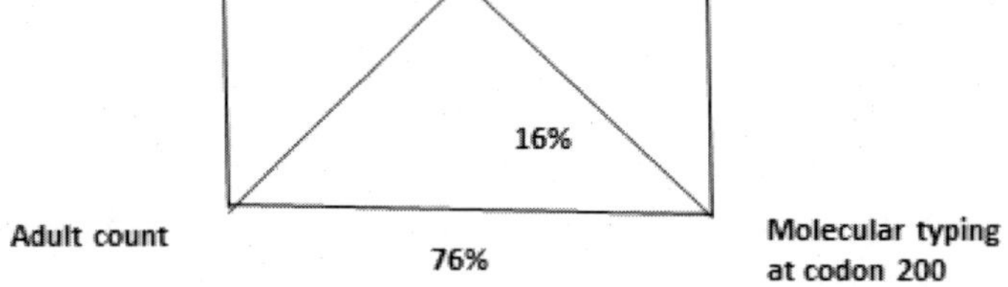

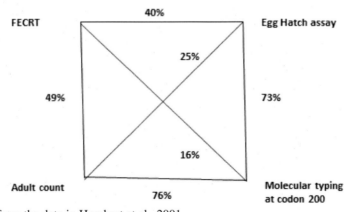

Drawn from the data in Humbert et al., 2001.

Figure 1. Phenotypic evaluations of anthelmintic resistance in gastro-intestinal nematodes of sheep and goats: FECRT with egg counts in faeces, egg hatch assay, adult worm count at necropsy, and molecular typing for resistance to benzimidazole. The highest percentage corresponds to the higher correlation between two measures of resistance.

The potential for detecting low level of resistance using molecular methods is only available for benzimidazoles, even if some markers could be used for an amino-acetonitrile derivative, monepantel (Kaminski et al., 2008) or possibly levamisole (Boulin et al., 2011) or other cholinergic agonist drugs (Charvet et al., 2012).

The genetic identification of resistance (available for benzimidazoles) requires fairly large samples (either adult worm or infective larvae). The probability of not finding resistant individuals, although they are present in a population, follows a hypergeometric distribution.

Thus the probability that tested worms are categorized as benzimidazole susceptible phenotype (SS and rS) is $(1-p)^n$, n being the number of worms tested and p the frequency of resistant worms (rr) in the population.

It is readily calculated that the number of worms to be processed in order to find at least one resistant individual is 100, 50, 35 and 20 for, respectively, 4%, 8%, 10% and 12% resistant genotypes in the population. Thus, as few as 100 individuals are needed to detect low level of resistance using a molecular marker.

The FECRT remains the most widely used test for detecting resistance in the different drugs, although, its sensitivity is not very good. The next chapter will investigate the sources of variation in FECRT in order to increase its accuracy for detecting resistance.

III. The Faecal Egg Count Reduction Test: Limiting Its Variability

Coles et al. (2006) presented the conditions for obtaining consistent results with FECRT sheep and goats (WAAVP): - Choose animals 3–6 months of age or, if older, with faecal eggs counts >150 epg.- Use 10 animals per group if possible.

- Count the eggs using the McMaster technique as soon as possible after collection.
- Individually weigh the animals and administer the manufacturers recommend dose of the anthelmintic.
- Take a second rectal faecal sample at the following time periods after treatment to count eggs:

Levamisole 3–7 days; Benzimidazole 8–10 days; Macrocyclic lactones 14–17 days; and if testing all groups in same flock, collect at 14 days. The variations in days after treatment are due to the different pharmacokinetics of the drugs. A 95% FEC reduction in ruminants and 90% reduction in horses based on arithmetic averages is expected in susceptible GIN populations or communi-ties. Based on the observed percentage reduction of FEC, the evaluation of anthelmintic efficacy using FECR are thus a means for defining the level of resistance. The VICH (http://www.vichsec.org/en/guidelines2.htm) guidelines to detect anthelmintic resistance were largely designed for use in experimental conditions based on worm counts after necropsy in ruminants. The evaluation of anthelmintic efficacy based on FECR was only presented for horses. In which case it recommends that there should be at least six test animals per group and the normal anthelmintic efficacy considered to be a 90% reduction based on geometric means of FEC. From these guidelines, we identified the following as potential sources of variation:

- a low level of EPG before treatment may preclude any conclusions
- the dosage and quality of a drug, particularly when generic drugs are used, is a prerequisite of an unbiased test
- the test period after treatment may vary according to the drug
- the efficacy may be based on arithmetic or geometric means depending on the distribution of FEC and the cut-off between susceptible and resistant communities to anthelmintics may vary from 90 to 95% depending on host species.

Only one formula for evaluating the efficacy of anthelmintics was used in the Coles et al. (1992) guidelines which compared the FEC in a treated and a control group after treatment. Later, different manners of calculating anthelmintic efficacy became available (Mejia et al., 2003; Torgerson et al., 2005; McKenna 2006) which yielded different values of efficacy. We will consider these sources of variation and how to control them.

a) Choosing the Right Animals and the Optimal Sample Size to Test for the Presence of Anthelmintic Resistance (Table 2 and 3)

The animals selected to be sampled for FECRT should have a sufficient level of EPG prior to treatment with anthelmintics.

Table 2. Anthelmintic efficacy (10 days after treatment) and confidence intervals of tetramisole or albendazole treatment in ewes with different level of initial EPG

EPG category (no of ewes sampled)	Drugs	
	Tetramisole	Albendazole
<300		
10	4 (0-24)[*]	53 (28-81)
15	4(0-16)	53 (33-80)
20	4 (0-8)	53 (30-74)
>300 and <600		
10	26 (5-50)	80 (44-95)
15	26 (7-48)	79 (55-94)
20	26 (9-44)	78 (60-94)
>600		
10	57 (27-76)	93 (69-100)
15	54 (32-73)	93 (79-100)
20	54 (35-69)	93 (78-99)

[*]Average anthelmintic efficacy in percentage and bootstrap 95% confidence interval.
Adapted from Cabaret and Berrag, 2004.

Table 3. FEC and faecal cultures after two treatments with albendazole (day 20), standard Dash et al. 1988 FECRT and Egg hatch assay-EHA (day 10)

Farm	Positive EPG after repeated treatment:	Positive larval cultures (genera) after repeated treatment	FECRT (Dash et al. 1988) after first treatment. (Yes= resistance)	EHA > 0.10 mg/ml Thiabendazole after first treatment (Yes= resistance)
1	Yes	Yes (Tela, Tricho)[*]	78 (Yes)	(No)
2	Yes	Yes (Tela, Tricho)	41 (Yes)	(Yes)
3	Yes	Yes (Tricho)	76 (Yes)	(No)
4	Yes	Yes (Tela, Tricho)	88 (Yes)	(No)
5	Yes	Yes (Tela, Tricho)	95 (No)	(No)

[*]Teladorsagia (Tela), Trichostrongylus (Tricho).
Adapted from Bentounsi et al., 2007.

A study was carried out to determine the efficacy of FECRT in relation to initial FEC to detect the presence of GIN resistance against tetramisole (a drug comparable to levamisole) and albendazole in a large sheep flock in Morocco (Table 2). Three different levels of EPG were defined within the flock, with 10 – 20 sheep subsamples randomly selected to represent each level. The EPG levels ranged from less than 300 to more than 600. The study highlighted several important points for consideration. Firstly, even when as many as 20 animals were sampled within a single EPG level, the bootstrap confidence intervals for the FECRT remained large showing that substantial variability remains between FECR estimations from the individual animals. We therefore suggest that 10 animals would constitute a representative sample size to reflect reductions in FEC as a result of anthelmintic treatment given the confidence interval was not greatly reduced with increasing numbers of animals.

Secondly, it is important to consider that the initial FEC prior to treatment has a strong influence on the estimation of tetramisole efficacy, which is found to increase in heavier infected animals.

Often the average EPG of a host is below 300, especially for GIN infections of cattle or ewes. In such cases, methods other than standard FECRT should be used. A variation of this test referred to as the repeated FECRT has been tested in ewes (Bentounsi et al., 2007: table 3). This involved a standard FECRT, where the FEC were performed on the first and tenth day after treatment with albendazole followed by another FECRT done 10 days after a second treatment with albendazole (Table 3). The GIN were found to be resistant except in farm five according to the standard FECRT. The repeated FECRT detected resistance in all farms.

The EHA detected resistance only in farm 2.

Further tests should be carried out on the repeated FECRT as they appear to be more sensitive to detect anthelmintic resistance in animals with low FEC.

b) Using the Right Dose and Drug

Many falsified drugs are available on informal markets (i.e., from the internet, small local providers in some countries, or poor quality generic drugs) which likely contribute to inaccurate estimations of anthelmtinic resistance (Cabaret, 2010). Furthermore even where approved drugs are used, under-dosing the animals is a frequent problem. An accurate estimate of the animal weight class is an important factor for the optimal metabolism of the anthelmintic.

Often, the weight is under-estimated by farmers judging by eye rather than with the use of scales. Finally, under-dosing may also result from the drench guns being poorly calibrated, and the drenching technique not always being fully mastered by the administrator (http://www.scops.org.uk/anthelmintics-treating-correctly.html). In such cases, the treatment failure is not always attributable to anthelmintic resistance.

Even with accurate dosing, approved generic drugs may also have poor efficacy against GIN infections (sheep: Wyk et al., 1997 in South Africa-rafoxanide, Bentounsi et al. 2003 in Algeria-albendazole, horse: Toscan et al., 2012-ivermectin). The physical properties of the generic drugs may vary largely even within the same drug class, as shown from an evaluation of albendazole drugs originating from Columbia, Guatemala, Peru and Thailand (Galia et al., 1999). In addition to the differing content and purity of the drug formulation, their ability to release the required amount of drugs within a certain time is an important factor in drug quality. Albendazole has low solubility and the release characteristics of the dosage play an important role in the availability of the drug, either in terms of systemic and/or local availability in the gut. The quality of excipients used in manufacturing of the drugs and the quality of the process itself is consequently of great importance to the performance of poorly soluble drugs such as albendazole.

A comparison of dissolution tests with albendazole from different manufacturers shows the release of their respective products varies largely, which likely has ramifications on the bioavailability of the active ingredients. The generic albendazoles also yield different efficacy results as shown from a study in Algerian sheep (Bentounsi et al., 2003). The study which tested six different generic albendazole drugs using the standard formula for FECRT (Dash et al. 1988), found their reductions to be 70, 71, 78 80, 89, and 93%.

The efficacy of another benzimidazole (innovator Fenbendazole) or a pro-benzimidazole (innovator Netobimin) was 92% in the same study. The significant following FECR groups were established fenbendazole, netobimin, two generic albendazoles, and four generic albendazoles, and untreated control. Thus four out of six generic albendazoles demonstrated lower efficacy than expected.

There are however many generic drugs of high quality with minimal differences detected between the innovator and the drug prepared by the initial manufacturer of the drug (Valdez et al., 1995 for pyrantel tartrate in horses, Mejia et al. 2003 for fenbendazole and ivermectin in cattle). It is therefore important to bear in mind the variability that exists in anthelmintic efficacy before making any hasty conclusions regarding the presence of resistance.

c) Choosing the Right Moment After Treatment to Check Anthelmintic Efficacy

The Coles et al. (2006) WAAVP recommendations proposed anthelmintic-specific post-treatment time lapses to verify their efficacy. A study by Lima et al. (2010) looked at the efficacy of different anthelmintics in goats (Table 4) over two seasons. The study found that: 1) the albendazole efficacy was overestimated at day 7 post-treatment; 2) the efficacy of ivermectin is highly variable on day 7 and 14 but stabilizes at day 21; 3) the efficacy of levamisole does not change much from day 7 to 21 post-treatment. A study into the anthelmintic FECR in European cattle GIN found that ivermectin efficacy could be estimated equally well on day 7, 14 or 21 post-treatment (Table 5).

Table 4. FECR using Coles et al. 1992 formula at various days after anthelmintic treatment in goats during the rainy and dry season in Brazil

Anthelmintic	Season	Post treatment efficacy		
		Day 7	Day 14	Day 21
Albendazole	Rainy	61	11	24
	Dry	55	14	12
Ivermectin	Rainy	14	70	66
	Dry	76	34	71
Levamisole	Rainy	89	79	73
	Dry	76	69	67

Data from Lima et al., 2010.

Table 5. FECR (average and range) of Ivermectin on GIN using before after formula - Kochapakdee et al. in 23 cattle farms from northern Europe

Gastro-intestinal nematodes groups based on FECR in % of drug	Post-treatment FECR on sampling days	
	Day 7/14	Day 21
Susceptible (FECR> or equal 95% on one of the sampling date) (8 farms)	95 (81-98)	95 (93-98)
Intermediate (7 farms)	96 (90-98)	90 (86-94)
Resistant (FECR<80% on one of the sampling) (8 farms)	87 (69-100)	63 (35-81)

Modified from Demeler et al., 2009.

Conversely, this efficacy was over-estimated at day 7 and 14 post-treatment in resistant GIN populations and was found to be better assessed on day 21 post-treatment. Despite the observed fluctuations in anthelmintic FECR throughout time, the presence of resistance was clear by day 14 post-treatment with the only uncertainty pertaining to the exact level of this resistance.

d) Which Formula Should Be Used to Calculate Anthelmintic Efficacy?

The FECRT provides an estimation of anthelmintic efficacy by comparing the worm egg counts from treated or non-treated hosts, before and after treatment show the reduction in infection level as a function of faecal egg counts. Although a standardised FECRT method (Coles et al., 2006) exists, several authors present their results having used several different methods: Kochapakdee et al. (1995) used four methods (Coles et al., 1992; Presidente, 1985, before and after treatment in treated hosts), Mejia et al. (2003) in cattle or Craven et al. (1998) in horses with five methods, Torres-Acosta et al., 2005 used "individual" and "average" methods, as if they could not decide which is the best adapted to their data.

There is therefore a need to evaluate the pros and cons for each method of FECRT. All the currently used methods are based on using the average of the sampled animals for calculating FECR. The average FECR may depend mostly on one or few animals. The individual response of hosts is thus highly informative; low efficacy results obtained in only a few hosts does not suggest anthelmintic resistance of the worm population, but rather indicates that the poor efficacy was due to either poor metabolism or availability of the drug in these animals. These are the reasons why two individually-based methods have been proposed (Cabaret and Berrag 2004): the FECRs are evaluated on each animal and then averaged.

The following formulas for estimating faecal egg count reduction are:

- based on averages: Presidente 1985, Dash et al. 1988, Kochapakdee et al. 1995, Coles et al. 1992,
- or individually based FECR (Cabaret and Berrag, 2004,) without a control group (iFECR3: before-after/before treatment, individual counterpart of Kochapakdee et al. 1995) and with a control group iFECR4 (individual counterpart of the assessments of Dash et al., 1988).

The average FECR (the reduction in EPG is evaluated on averages of the groups) were calculated as follows (FECR nomenclature as in Mejia et al., 2003; Cabaret, 2004):

1 Presidente, 1985: FECR5=(100x (1-[T2/T1] [C1/C2] (geometric average),
2 Dash et al., 1988: FECR4=(100x (1-[T2/T1]) [C1/C2] (arithmetic average). This corresponds to the Henderson and Tilton (1955) formula used for toxicity in insects.
3 Kochapakdee et al., 1995: FECR3=(100x (1-[T2/T1] (arithmetic average),
4 Coles et al., 2003: FECR1=(100x (1-[T2/C2] (arithmetic average). It corresponds to the Abbott (1925) formula used for toxicity in insects.Where C = control groups; T = treated groups; 1 = D0; 2 = D10. The Coles et al. (1992) 95% confidence interval was established using the RESO© method (CSIRO 1990 Animal Health Division).
5 Mejia et al. 2003: FECR is based on general linear model (GLM) where the EPG after treatment may be evaluated in relation to the initial EPG, taking into account other variables such as age of animal, dosage etc. Estimated means (means corrected for the other factors of variation) are then obtained and these means (instead of arithmetic or geometric means) serve for evaluated the FECR.

The individually based FECR are calculated according to Cabaret and Berrag 2004: iFECR3=(100x (1-[T2/T1]; iFECR4 =(100x (1-[T2/T1]) [C1/ C2] (calculated on individual sample values and then averaged for the group).

The FECR is calculated on individual values in each group and the FECR values are then averaged.

Below is an example to illustrate the differences between average and individual-based estimation of FECR.

Five animals (a-e) in a treatment group were tested on Day 0 and Day 10 post-treatment (iFECR3 and FECR3). The respective FEC were as follows

- Day 0: a = 100, b = 200, c = 700, d = 450, e = 300 EPG. Average for treatment group = 350 EPG.
- Day 10: a = 50, b = 0, c = 250, d = 0, e = 0 EPG. Average for treatment group = 60 EPG.
- FECR4= (350-60)/60= 58%

- iFECR4= [(100-50)/100+(200-0)/200+ (700-250)/700 + (450-0)/450) + (300-0)/300]/5= 82.8%

In this example the two values are very different, due to the failure of treatment in two of the animals (a and c) and FECR should be taken with caution since it is related to the particular efficacy in only two animals.

The inclusion of an untreated control on day 0 and day 10-12 post treatment (FECR4, FECR5, iFECR4, Mejia et al. 2003) is a real advantage for the estimation of FECR for all these methods as the EPG could evolve within this 10 day period. Given the additional costs associated with this extra FEC (i.e., sampling time, the larger number of faecal egg counts processed) it explains why other methods were proposed.

For example, the Coles et al. (1992) procedure uses samples of an untreated control and a treated group, but only on day 10 after treatment.

The authors for the various FECR formulas used a threshold to determine anthelmintic efficacy ranging from 90% (Presidente, 1985, Dash et al., 1988, Kochakapdee et al., 1995), to 95% (Coles et al., 1992; Coles et al., 2006). The present cut-off values for diagnosing resistance are not based on any solid investigation and in future it would be needed to have sound cut-off values.

The main problem of these FECR is that we do not have any confidence intervals, except for the Coles et al. (1992) formula. We propose bootstrap resampling to obtain 95% confidence intervals for both the individual and average FECR estimations. There are currently two software programs that can do this which are available for free on demand to the authors (Resivers-Cabaret and Berrag, 2004 for individual, and Bootstreat- Cabaret and Antoine, 2008 for average estimates of FECR).

Individual versus Average Methods

A comparison of these individual and average methods (from Cabaret and Berrag, 2004 presented in Table 6)found major discrepancies in 4 out of 16 farms constituting a nearly 30% difference in FECR. The discrepancies were not related on the basis of initial EPG, host species, or level of efficacy, but instead they were related to the presence of few animals presenting highly different FECR from the rest of the group.

Animals with different responses to treatment should be checked again for treatment efficacy, before concluding that the existence of anthelmintic resistance is present. The individual estimation of FECR can be calculated with a confidence interval at p=0.95 using bootstrap resampling procedure (free software available on demand to the author).

Table 6. Comparative faecal egg count reduction test using individual and average methods. Main discrepancies with figures in bold

Data origin and anthelminthic	Individual evaluation		Average evaluation	
	iFECR3	iFECR4	FECR3	FECR4
Morocco (Sheep)				
Albendazole	87	76	97	97
Tetramisole	38	27	37	30
Algeria (sheep)				
Albendazole	**36**	**37**	**71**	**71**
Albendazole	91	90	86	93
Albendazole	80	80	82	80
Albendazole	90	81	89	89
Albendazole	**40**	**42**	**69**	**70**
Albendazole	59	77	78	78
Netobimin	89	83	92	92
Fenbendazole	89	88	92	92
Argentina (cattle)				
Fenbendazole	67	51	67	67
Fenbendazole	49	45	36	37
Ivermectin	89	84	92	92
Ivermectin	89	90	87	87
Fenbendazole	**65**	**46**	**80**	**87**
Ivermectin	**91**	**84**	**50**	**66**

Adapted from Cabaret and Berrag, 2004.

Average Methods and General Model Estimates

The different formulas are in acceptable agreement in sheep GIN infections (table 7) where high levels of efficacy are attained. However, the results indicate an absence of resistance to albendazole with the Coles et al. (1996) formula whereas resistance was clearly identified using the formula of Mejia et al. (2003) based on a classical general model analysis of variance. The same finding was presented for cattle by Mejia et al., 2013: the FECR was 92% effective using the average methods and 80% effective with the Mejia et al. method. The apparent convergence should not be over-interpreted since it may lead to different conclusions on resistance in the field to thereby alter significantly the choice of anthelmintics to be used.

The FECR are again somewhat in the same range when medium (70 to 85%) to low efficacy (less than 70%) are considered (Table 8), although very different efficacies have been recorded in some instances (see Alb1 from 8 to 49%; Ive1 with 65 to 81%).

Table 7. Comparison of several FECRT methods when drug efficacy is high

	Anthelmintic			
Methods for calculating FECR	Albendazole	Fenbendazole	Netobimin	Ivermectin
Coles et al.	95	92	95	100
Kochapakdee et al.	86	92	92	100
Dash et al.	93	92	92	100
Mejia et al.	85	93	92	99

Adapted from Bentounsi et al., 2003.

Table 8. Comparison of several FECRT methods when drug efficacy is medium to low

Method for calculating FECR	Goat			Cattle			
	Alb1	Alb2	Lev	Fen1	Fen2	Ive1	Ive2
Coles et al.	11	70	83	31	61	80	54
Kochapakdee et al.	49	77	85	36	67	80	50
Dash et al.	8	58	81	37	67	87	65
Presidente	ND	ND	ND	67	79	89	77
Mejia et al.	ND	ND	ND	41	51	65	47

Alb: albendazole, Lec: levamisole, Fen: fenbendazole, Ive: ivermectin; ND: not done. Modified from Lima et al., 2010 and Mejia et al., 2003.

This may alter treatment decisions. Some may interpret a 70 to 85% efficacy as a sufficient level to justify the continued use of a drug for a limited time (van Wyk, 2009 personal communication), even in the knowledge that resistance may increase.

Whereas others may abandon a drug with low or very low efficacy and turn to other drugs, or combinations of drugs.

Guerrero et al. (2010) analysed the FECR obtained by Craven et al. (1998) in horses and found that the consistency between these methods was strong at high efficacy but poor at low efficacy, in particular for the formula of Presidente (1985) (Table 9). The most used method (before/after treatment) was significantly correlated (Spearmann coefficient between 0.65 to 0.78) to other methods when the efficacy was higher than 90% (and then GIN are considered as susceptible.

Table 9. Spearman correlation between efficacy before after/treatment (Kochapakdee et al.) and other calculation methods in horses

	FECR according to Kochapakdee et al.		
	.>90% (n=42)	Between 70% and 90% (n=15)	<70% (n=15)
Coles et al.	**0.74**	**0.66**	0.31
Dash et al.	**0.78**	**0.61**	-0.01
Presidente	**0.65**	0.12	-0.03

Adapted from Guerrero et al., 2010. Correlations in bold are significant at $p<0.05$.

These correlations mean that in the best case, the coefficient of explanation was 0.64 (i.e., [coefficient of correlation]^2= 0.78^2) meaning that many farms will be categorized incorrectly as resistant or not resistant to anthelmintics.

Determining the best method to measure the onset of resistance differs from determining the level of established anthelmintic resistance. Where a new anthelmintic is used, or when no resistance has been demonstrated on a specific farm, the efficacy estimated by faecal egg count reduction (FECR) is likely to be very close to 100%. The sustainability of anthelmintics will depend on our capacity to detect departure from 100% efficacy. Dobson et al. 2012 proposed a method for this detection. A novel way to determine the lower confidence limit for 100% efficacy is to reframe FECR as a binomial proportion, i.e., define: n and x as the total number of eggs counted (rather than eggs per gram of faeces) for all pre-treatment and post-treatment animals, respectively. The proportion of resistant eggs is $p= x/n$ and percent efficacy is $100 \times (1 - p)$ (assuming equal treatment group sizes and detection levels, before and after treatment).

Dobson et al. 2012 indicated that for 100% efficacy at least 37 eggs need to be counted pre-treatment before the lower confidence interval can exceed 90%. This means that 37 eggs are counted and that in the most usual case (a sensitivity to 50 eggs per gram) and thus 37 x 50= 1850 EPG are required which is not so frequent in a large number of infections.

Composite Versus Individual Faecal Samples

Composite FEC have also been used to assess the level of infestation by GIN in sheep (Morgan et al., 2005). McKenna (2007) suggested that the use of composite FEC could also be used to establish the efficacy of anthelmintics, although, it has rarely been used in the field (Jones et al., 2010 in sheep or Guerrero et al. 2010 in horses).

Table 10. Efficacy of fenbendazole in horses using before/after treatment estimates either on individually sampled animals or on a composite faecal sample collected from the ground

Tested horses	Average efficacy on individual samples	Composite efficacy	Conclusion on resistance for both evaluations
Older foals (38 animals with 50% uninfected)	55	-96	Yes
Yearlings (nine animals, all infected)	50	Estimate one:5%	Yes
		Estimate two 12%:	Yes

Modified from Guerrero et al. 2010.

Studies showed the estimation of anthelmintic efficacy in horses with use of composite FEC was mediocre in terms of efficacy values (<90% corresponding to resistance), but indicative in both cases of resistance to benzimidazoles (Table 10).

A simulation (Calvete and Uriarte, 2013) showed that a sample composite was one of the best FECR estimates when based on the Coles et al. (1992) formula. However, this was not the most practical option. Given the faeces are collected on pasture and the treated and the control groups would likely graze together, it would be difficult to attribute the faecal sample to one group or another. This could be made easier with use of sheep pens in which the animals could be separated into treated or untreated groups prior to the collection of faeces from the ground. The simulation study further showed that the number of FEC conducted on a single composite was relatively high (up to 20), and thereby reduced the interest of using the method via increased laboratory costs. For farmers, the easiest diagnostic is based on composite FEC, before and after treatment, without a control group, but it was less efficient in the evaluating of FECR. The use of composite FEC to monitor the efficacy of anthelmintics needs improvement, but nonetheless it appears to be able to indicate the gross value of FECR and probably permits the detection of high level of resistance in most cases. The diversity of possible evaluations of anthelmintic efficacy, and their results, makes it difficult to decide upon the optimum use of anthelmintics in a specific farm situation. We thus propose a tentative strategy to decide upon an anthelmintic treatment plan.

Conclusion: Tentative Proposals for Improved Practices Using FECRT and Anthelmintic Treatment Decisions

Firstly, it is important to determine the level of resistance on a farm to both old and new anthelmintics. The management of anthelmintic resistance cannot be set apart from the husbandry choices of the farm owner or the shepherd (Saddiqui et al., 2012). The second step is then to have a diagnostic on the intensity of infection. It would be useful to do this for both the younger and older animals on the farm using composite FEC. This should then be followed up with diagnostics for the presence of anthelmintic resistance against the commonly used drugs. This could be done with a single post-treatment FEC carried out between day 10 to 14. If the FECs are found to be high and the herd/flock presents other symptoms of GIN infection such as anaemia, diarrhea, cachexia or diminished production traits, then action should be taken to reduce the GIN (or fluke, or other) infection. The choice of the anthelmintic is then very important. Clearly, it should have efficiency against the targeted parasites. The use of anthelmintics with already limited activity (60 to 80% resistance) could be used or discarded. For example, in resource poor farming limited efficacy anthelmintics may be selected for use if the cost is low (levamisole for example), or if resistance to other anthelmintics is already present given it will confer partial protection in the most heavily infected animals in need of treatment. This solution would be largely limited in time as resistance to the drug increased. This would require consistent surveying of the real efficacy of the anthelmintic throughout time. In cases where economic resources are more readily available, the use of anthelmintics which already have resistance against them should be avoided, and another anthelmintic selected for use. If multi-drug resistance is an issue, then the combination of several drugs is the only solution. These high resistance situations have resulted from inappropriate management of GIN. The vast majority of farms continue to rely upon anthelmintic treatment as their sole means for controlling GIN infection. This does not represent a sustainable management strategy as new drugs are rarely delivered onto the market. Instead, high and multi-anthelmintic resistance situations should be controlled using integrated management techniques such as pasture management (rotation, mixed species grazing etc.) against parasite transmission stages and to further consider the switch to using animals breeds or genotypes with less susceptibility, or greater resilience to infection.

Checking anthelmintic resistance status' is thus an absolute necessity before undertaking any kind of appropriate management of GIN infection.

There is a real need for easy and low cost methods to detect anthelmintic resistance. Composite faecal sampling in all host species could be a good solution for estimating the gross situation of infection however, there is a need to better calibrate this technique. Presently, the Dash et al. (1988) formula is the best to assess efficacy. It takes into account the evolution of EPG in a control group and in a treated group. However this also represents a potentially costly option as it requires sampling of 10 animals on days 0 and 10 post-treatment meaning a minimum of 40 FEC need to be sent to a laboratory for testing against a single anthelmintic.

This evaluation would not however be needed frequently, but required before building a plan to manage GIN properly.

Acknowledgments

The comments on the manuscript and improvement of the English by Caroline Chylinski (INRA, Nouzilly) are gratefully acknowledged. This paper was originally inspired from the discussions with many colleagues in the Strep (Drastic and Sustainable Treatment Reduction against Parasitism in livestock) research program funded by the Integrated Management of Animal Health - INRA Animal Health Department.

References

Abbott, W. S. (1925). A method of computing the effectiveness of an insecticide. *J. Econ. Entomol.*, 18, 265-267.

Barnes, E. H., Dobson, R. J., Barger, I. A. (1995). Worm control and anthelmintic resistance: adventures with a model. *Parasitol. Today* 11, 56-63.

Barrere, V., Falzon, L. C., Shakya, K. P., Menzies, P. I., Peregrine, A. S., Prichard, R. K. (2013)., Assessment of benzimidazole resistance in *Haemonchus contortus* in sheep flocks ∗in Ontario, Canada: Comparison of detection methods for drug resistance. *Vet. Parasitol.* 198 (2013) 159–165.

Bentounsi, B., Attir, B., Meradi, S., Cabaret, J. (2007). Repeated treatment faecal egg counts to identify gastrointestinal nematode resistance in a context of low-level infection of sheep on farms in eastern Algeria. *Vet. Parasitol.* 144, 104–110.

Bentounsi, B., Zouiouech, H., Benchikh-Elfegoun, C., Kohil, K., Bouzekri, M., Cabaret, J. (2003). Efficacité comparée des spécialités d'Albendazole distribués en Algérie. *Rev. Med. Vét.* 154, 649-652.

Boulin, T., Fauvin, A., Charvet, C., Cortet, J., Cabaret, J., Bessereau, J. L., Neveu, C. (2011). Functional Reconstitution of *Haemonchus contortus* Acetylcholine Receptors in *Xenopus* Oocytes Provides Mechanistic Insights into Levamisole Resistance. *Brit. J. Pharmacol.*, 164, 1421-1432.

Buxton, S. K., Charvet, C. L., Neveu, C., Cabaret, J., Cortet, J., Peineau, N., Abongwa, M., Courtot, E., Peineau, N., Robertson, A. P., Martin, R. J. (2014) Investigation of Acetylcholine Receptor Diversity in a Nematode Parasite Leads to Characterization of Tribendimidine- and Derquantel-Sensitive nAChRs. *PLoS Pathog.* 10(1): e1003870. doi:10.1371/journal.ppat.1003870.

Coles, G. C., Bauer, C., Borgsteed, F. H. M., Geerts, D., Klei, T. R., Taylor, M. A., Waller, P. J. (1992). World association for the advancement of veterinary parasitology (WAAVP) methods for the detection of anthelmintic resistance in nematodes of veterinary importance. *Vet. Parasitol.*, 1992, 44, 35-44.

Coles, G. C., Jackson, F., Pomroy, W. E., Prichard, R. K., von Samson-Himmelstjerna, G., Silvestre, A., Taylor, M. A., Vercruysse, J. (2006). The detection of anthelmintic resistance in nematodes of veterinary importance. *Vet. Parasitol.* 136, 167–185.

Cabaret, J. (2004). Efficacy evaluation of anthelmintics: which methods to use in the field? *Parassitologia*, 46, 241-243.

Cabaret, J., (2010). False Resistance to Antiparasitic Drugs: Causes from Shelf Availability to Patient Compliance. *Anti-Infect. Agents Med. Chem.*, 9, 161-167.

Cabaret, J., Antoine, T. (2008). The two main problems in evaluating resistance to antiparasitic drugs in populations of naturally infected hosts: efficacy variability and cut-off value for resistance. *Proceedings Ehrlich II, 2nd World Conference on Magic ballets*. Nürnberg, Germany, October.

Cabaret, J., Berrag, B. (2004). Faecal egg count reduction test for assessing anthelmintic efficacy: average versus individually based estimations. *Vet. Parasitol.* 121, 105–113.

Cabaret, J., Silvestre, A. Management of nematode infection and resistance against anthelminthics: Towards a sustainable control in herbivores. In: *Nematodes: Morphology, Functions and Management Strategies*. Boeri,

F. and J. A. Chung Ed. New York (US): Nova Science Publishers, 2012.- 179-196. ISBN: 978-1-61470-784-4 (Animal Science, Issues and Professions).

Calvete, C., Uriarte, J. (2013) Improving the detection of anthelmintic resistance: Evaluation of faecal egg count reduction test procedures suitable for farm routines. *Vet. Parasitol.*, 196, 438-452.

Charvet, C. L., Robertson, A. P., Cabaret, J., Martin, R. J., Neveu, C. (2012). Selective effect of the anthelmintic bephenium on *Haemonchus contortus* levamisole-sensitive acetylcholine receptors. *Invert. Neurosci.*, 12: 43-51.

Craven, J., Bjorn, H., Henriksen, S. A., Nansen, P., Larsen, M., Lendal, S. (1998). Survey of anthelmintic resistance on Danish horse farms, using 5 different methods of calculating faecal egg count reduction. *Equine Vet. J.,* 30, 289-293.

Cudekova, P., Varady, M., Dolinska, M., Konigova, A. (2010). Phenotypic and genotypic characterisation of benzimidazole susceptible and resistant isolates of *Haemonchus contortus. Vet. parasitol.*, 172, 155-159.

Dash, K., Hall, K., Barger, I. A. (1988). The role of arithmetic and geometric worm egg counts in faecal egg count reduction test and in monitoring strategic drenching programs in sheep. *Aust. Vet.* 65, 66-68.

Demeler, J., Van Zeveren, A. M. J., Kleinschmidt, N., Vercruysse, J., Höglund, J., Koopmann, R., Cabaret, J., Claerebout, E., G. von Samson-Himmelstjerna, E. G. (2009). Monitoring the efficacy of ivermectin and albendazole against gastro intestinal nematodes of cattle in Northern Europe. *Vet. Parasitol.*, 160: 109-115.

Dobson, R., Hosking, B., Jacobson, C., Cotter, J., Besier, R., Stein, P., Reid, S. (2012). Preserving new anthelmintics: a simple method for estimating faecal egg count reduction test (FECRT) confidence limits when efficacy and/or nematode aggregation is high. *Vet. Parasitol.* 186, 79–92.

Duncan, J. L., Abbott, E. M., Arundel, J. H., Eysker, M., Klei, T. R., Krecek, R. C., Lyons, E. T., Reinemeyer, C., Slocombe, J. O. D. (2002). World association for the advancement of veterinary parasitology (WAAVP): second edition of guidelines for evaluating the efficacy of equine anthelmintics. *Vet. Parasitol.*, 103, 1-18.

Elard, L., Cabaret, J., Humbert, J. F. (1999). PCR diagnosis of benzimidazole-susceptibity or -resistance in natural populations of the small ruminant parasite, *Teladorsagia circumcincta. Vet. Parasitol.*, 80, 231–237.

Guerrero, M. C., Duchamp, G., Reigner, F., Cabaret, J. (2010). La résistance des strongles aux anthelminthiqueschez les équins: mesure simplifiée par des échantillons composites. p.103-108. *Proceedings, 36ème Journées de la Recherche Equine*, Paris.

Galia, E., Horton, J., Dressman, B. (1999). Albendazole generics- Acomparative in vitro study. *Pharm. Res.*, 16, 1871-1875.

Henderson, C. F., Tilton, E. W. (1955). Tests with acaricides against the brow wheat mite. *J. Econ. Entomol.* 48, 157-161.

Humbert, J. F., Cabaret, J., Elard, L., Leignel, V., Silvestre, A., 2001. Molecular approaches to studying benzimidazole resistance in trichostron-gylid nematode parasites of small ruminants. *Vet. Parasitol.* 101, 405-414.

Jones, J., Pearson, R., Jeckel, S. (2012). Suspected anthelmintic resistance to macrocyclic lactones in lambs in the UK. *Vet. Rec.*, 170, 59–60.

Kaminsky, R., Ducray, P., Jung, M., Clover, R., Rufener, L., Bouvier, J., Weber, S. S., Schorderet, S., Wenger, A., Wieland-Berghausen, S., Goebel, T., Gauvry, N., Pautrat, F., Skripsky, T., Froelich, O., Komoin-Oka, C., Westlund, B., Sluder, A., Maser, P. (2008). A new class of anthelmintics effective against drug-resistant nematodes. *Nature*, 452, 176-U19.

Kochapakdee, S., Pandey, V. S., Pralomkarm, W., Choldumrongkul, S., Ngampongsai, W., Lawpetchara, A., (1995). Anthelmintic resistance in goats in southern Thailand. *Vet. Rec.* 137, 124-125.

Martin, P. J., Anderson, N., Jarrett, G. (1989). Detecting benzimidazole resistance with faecal egg count reduction tests and in vitro assays. *Aust. Vet. J.* 66, 236–240.

Mejia, M. F., Fernandez Iguarta, B. M., Schmidt, E. E., Cabaret, J. (2003). Multispecies and multiple anthelminthic resistance on cattle nematodes in a farm in Argentina: the beginning of high resistance? *Vet. Res.* 34, 461-467.

McKenna, P. B. (2006). Further comparison of faecal egg count reduction test procedures: sensitivity and specificity. *N.Z. Vet. J.*, 54, 365–366.

McKenna, P. B. (2007).) How do you mean? The case for composite faecal egg counts in testing for drench resistance. *N. Z. Vet. J.*, 55, 100–101.

Mooney, L., Good, B., Hanrahan, J. P., Mulcahy, G., de Waal, T. (2009). The comparative efficacy of four anthelmintics against a natural acquired *Fasciola hepatica* infection in hill sheep flock in the west of Ireland. *Vet. Parasitol.*, 164, 201–205.

Kaplan, R. M. (2004). Drug resistance in nematodes of veterinary importance: a status report. *Trends Parasitol.* 20, 477-481.

Lima, W. C., Ahaide, A. C. R., Medeiros, G. R., Lima, D. A. S. D., Borburema, J. B., Santos, E. M., Vilela, V. L. R., Azevedo, S. S. (2010).

Nematoides resistentes a alguns anti-helminticos en rebanhos Caprinos no Cariri Paraibano. *Pesq. Brasileiras*, 30, 1003-1009.

Morgan, E. R., Cavill, L., Curry, G. E., Wood, R., Mitchell, E. S. E. (2005). Effects of aggregation and sample size on composite faecal egg counts in sheep. *Vet. Parasitol.*, 131, 79–87.

National Sheep Association (UK). Scops: Sustainable control of parasites in sheep http://www.scops.org.uk/anthelmintics-treating-correctly.html Accessed on the 5th of February 2014.

Olaechea, F., Lovera, V., Larroza, M., Raffo, F., Cabrera, R. (2011). Resistance of *Fasciola hepatica* against triclabendazole in cattle in Patagonia (Argentina). *Vet. Parasitol.*, 178, 364–366.

Overend, D. J., Phillips, M. L., Poulton, A. L., Foster, C. E. D., (1994). Anthelmintic resistance in Australian sheep nematode populations. *Aust. Vet. J.,* 71, 117-121.

Presidente, P. J. A., (1985). Methods for detection of resistance to anthelmintics. In: Anderson, N., Waller, P. J. (Eds), *Resistance in nematodes to anthelmintics.* CSIRO Division animal health, Glebe NSW, Australia p. 13-28.

Robertson, A. P., Buxton, S. K., Puttachary, S., Williamson, S. M., Wolstenholme, A. J., Neveu, C., Cabaret, J., Charvet, C. L., Martin, R. J. Antinematodal Drugs - Modes of Action and Resistance: And Worms Will Not Come to Thee (Shakespeare: Cymbeline: IV, ii). In: *Parasitic Helminths: Targets, Screens, Drugs and Vaccines.* Caffey, C. R. Ed. Weinheim (DEU): Wiley-Blackwell, 2012.- 233-249. ISBN: 978-3-527-33059-1 (Drug Discovery in Infectious Diseases).

Scott, I., Pomroy, W. E., Kenyon, P. R., Smith, G., Adlington, B., Moss, A. (2013). Lack of efficacy of monepantel against *Teladorsagia circumcincta* and *Trichostrongylus colubriformis*. *Vet. Parasitol.* 198, 166-171.

Silvestre, A., Leignel, V., Berrag, B., Gasnier, N., Humbert, J. F., Chartier, C., Cabaret, J., 2002, Sheep and goat nematode resistance to anthelmintics: pro and cons among breeding management factors. *Vet. Res.* 33, 465-480.

Saddiqi, H. A., Jabbar, A., Babar, W., Sarwar, M., Iqbal, Z., Cabaret, J. (2012). Contrasting views of animal healthcare providers on worm control practices for sheep and goats in an arid environment. *Parasite*, 19, 53-61.

Toscan, G., Cezar, A. S., Pereira, R. C. F., Silva, G. B., Sangioni, L. A., Oliveira, L. S. S., Vogel, F. S. F. (2012). Comparative performance of macrocyclic lactones against large strongyles in horses. *Parasitol. Int.* 61, 550-553.

Torgerson, P. R., Schnyder, M., Hertzberg, H. (2005). Detection of anthelmintic resistance: a comparison of mathematical techniques. *Vet. Parasitol.* 128, 291-298.

Torres-Acosta, J. F. J., Aguilar-Caballero, A. J., Le Bigot, C., Hoste, H., Canul-Ku, H. L., Santos-Ricalde, R., Gutierrez-Segura, I. (2005). Comparing different formulae to test for gastrointestinal nematode resistance to benzimidazoles in smallholder goat farms in Mexico. *Vet. Parasitol.* 134, 241-248.

Valdez, R. A., DiPietro, J. A., Paul, A. J., Lock, T. F., Hungerford, L. L., Tod, K. S. (1995). Controlled efficacy study of the bioequivalence of Strongid C and generic pyrantel tattrate in horses. *Vet. Parasitol.* 60, 83-102.

VICH Guidelines http://www.vichsec.org/en/guidelines2.htm (consulted the 3rd of February 2014).

Wyk, J. A. v., Stenson, M. O., Van der Merwe, J. S., Vorster, R. J., Viljoen, P. G., (1999). Anthelmintic resistance in South Africa: surveys indicate an extremely serious situation in sheep and goat farming. *Onderstepoort J. Vet. Res.*, 66, 273-284.

Wyk, J. A. v., Malan, F. S., van Rensburg, L. J., Oberem, P. T., M. J. Allan, M. J. (1997). Quality control in generic anthelmintics: Is it adequate? *Vet. Parasitol.* 72, 157-165.

In: Anthelmintics
Editor: William Quick
ISBN: 978-1-63117-714-9

Chapter 2

Anthelmintics: Clinical Pharmacology and Uses in Human and Veterinary Medicine

Ranjita Shegokar[1,*], Ph.D., Rajani Athawale[2], Ph.D. and Darshana Jain[2]

[1] Free University of Berlin, Department of Pharmaceutics, Biopharmaceutics and NutriCosmetics, Berlin, Germany

[2] C.U. Shah College of Pharmacy, SNDT University, Mumbai, India

Abstract

Anthelmintics are commonly used to treat parasitic worm infections in human and animals. These parasitic worms infect crops, domestic pets and livestock. Helminth, being tropical infectious disease gets less attention from developed world. The main chemotherapeutic agents used in humans are mainly adapted from veterinary medicine. Among them only few drugs have a broad spectrum activity while many drugs have very limited action against particular species. The few parameters like dosing frequency of anthelmintics, efficacy of drug, degree of infection

* Corresponding author: Ranjita Shegokar. Free University of Berlin, Department of Pharmaceutics, Biopharmaceutics and NutriCosmetics, Kelchstr. 31, 12169 Berlin, Germany. E-mail: ranjita@arcsindia.com.

and untreated population of parasitic worms in body affects the possibility of deve-lopping resistance both in human and animals.

However, various academics institutes and industry are working on new ways and the types of drug delivery systems for anthelmintic drugs. In this chapter, the current chemotherapy in veterinary and human medicine is reviewed. A detailed discussion on new drugs, formulation systems and clinical trial status is done at the end of chapter. The role of herbal antihelmintics is also discussed in detail. Special focus on the efficacy of various anthelmintic drugs in animals and human is given and debated.

Keywords: Anthelmintics, veterinary medicine, human medicine, pharmacology, drug delivery systems

Helmintic Infections in Human

Introduction

Background on Helmintics

"Helmint" means worm. The helminths are either elongated, flat or round worms. Approximately, 140,000 deaths are recorded each year due to soil transmitted helmintic infections (STH). They are mainly classified based on their external shape and/or the host organ on which they inhabit. Helminth exists in both hermaphroditic and bisexual species. Matured flukes are leaf-shaped flatworms and also called as trematodes. Flukes are hermaphroditic except for blood flukes, they are bisexual. The life-cycle includes a snail intermediate host. Adult tapeworms (flat worms/cestodes) are elongated, segmented, hermaphroditic flatworms that inhabit in an intestinal lumen. Larval forms, which are cystic or solid, inhabit in extra intestinal tissues (Figure 1). The mature and larval roundworms (nematodes) are bisexual, cylindrical worms. Males are usually smaller than females. The developmental process in nema-todes involves egg, larval, and adult stages, thereby completing full life cycle.

Helmintic infections occur in the intestinal tract, urinary tract, respiratory tract or blood of humans by schistosomes, intestinal nematodes (or soil-transmitted helminths, STH), and tissue nematodes, including human filariae that causes lymphaticfilariasis and onchocerciasis [1].

These groups are subdivided for convenience according to the host organ in which they reside, e.g., lung flukes, extra intestinal tapeworms, and intestinal roundworms. The complete understanding of life cycle of helminthes gives us an idea about their origin, pathogenesis, diagnosis and eventually treatment.

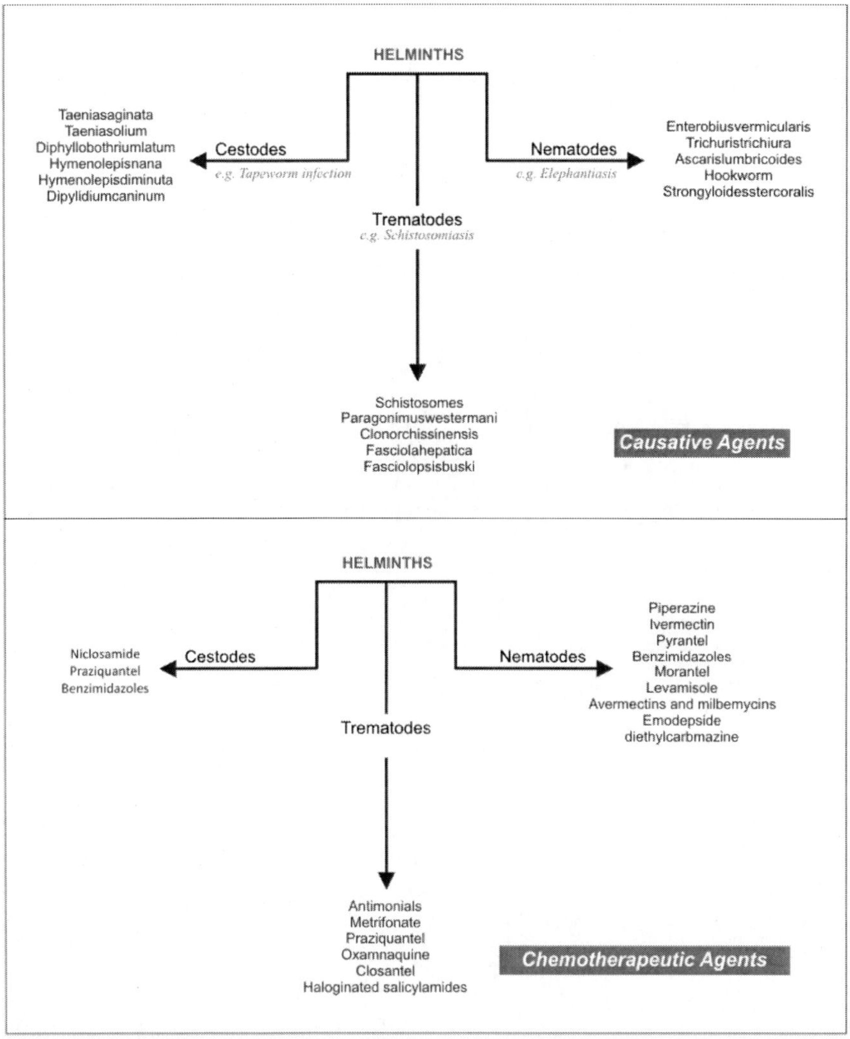

Figure 1. Type of helmintic infections in human and their causative agents (above) chemotherapy used to treat infections caused by cestodes, nematodes and trematodes (below).

Mainly hermaphroditic species of flukes and tapeworm infects human. Hermaphroditic flukes include *Clonorchis sinensis*, *Fasiolopsis buski, Parago-*

nimys westermani, and *Heterophytes heterpphyes.* Some bisexual flukes like *Schistosoma japonicum, S mansoni,* and *S hematobium* are also included in the list of infective flukes in human along with Cercariae and Metacercaria. A fluke, parasitic trematodes can transmit intact human skin and enter the capillaries and then migrate to the central system.

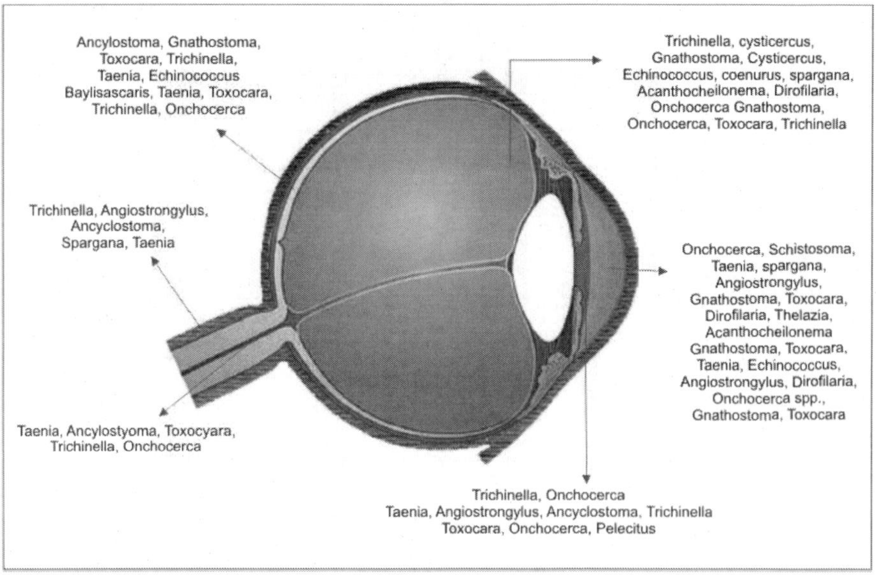

Figure 2. Helmintic infections of ocular system.

Acute schistosomiasis is also called as Katayama fever. Worldwide 250 species of capillaria are found among which only three are infectious to human. Helminthes also infects respiratory tract (Table 1), genital organs, ear and ocular systems. Figure 2 shows types of helmintic species and site of infection of ocular system.

Background of Anthelmintics

Anthelmintics are used to treat helmintic infections. A large human population harbors one to several species of helminths. In few cases, helminths lives in harmony with human body but in many cases they cause life threatening problems.

The form of anthelmintic treatment mainly depends on the type of infection, severity of infection and the site of infection. Among helmintic, STH infections affects majority of population to greater extent with very few treatment options available. Some intestinal forms include infection by tapeworms, including Taenia species.

Tissue forms include trematodes or flukes which causes schistosomiasis or bilharziasis. The drugs that treat fluke infections by *Schistosoma mansoni, S. japonicum and S. haematobium* are called antischistosomes. The anthelmintic treatment varies with the stage of the life cycle of parasite and age of patient.

Table 1. Helmintic infections of human respiratory system

Causative agent	Host	Method of infection
Schistosoma mansoni *Schistosoma haematobium* *Schistosoma japonicum* *Schistosoma intercalatum* *Schistosoma mekoni*	Human	Transdermal penetration
Necator americanus	Human	Transdermal penetration
Strongyloides stercoralis *Strongyloides fuellerborni*	Human	Transdermal penetration by larva autoinfection
Ancylostoma duodenale	Human	Transdermal penetration by larva
Ascaris lumbricoides	Human	Ingestion of eggs by water/food mode
Wuchereria bancrofti *Brugia malayi*	Human	Infection insect bite
Trichinella spiralis *Trichinella Nativa* *Trichinella Britovi* *Trichinella nelsoni*	Human	Injection of infected uncooked meat

The drugs available for human treatment were first developed as veterinary medicines. The use of praziquantel (for schistosomes) and albendazole or mebendazole (for STH) for helmintic infections is recommended by the World Health Organization (WHO).

Alternatively, the two nicotinic acetylcholine receptor (nAChR) agonist pyrantel and levamisole are also used in many instances. The continuous use of anthelmintics induces toxicity in humans and animals. Hence, the development and discovery of new chemical entities acting as anthelmintics are being synthesized and some of them are also derived from plants.

To exert action, anthelmintic drugs penetrate to the body of the worm by damage to the worm, causing paralysis, narcosis, or damaging its cuticle. Some anthelmintic drugs interfere with the metabolism, and disturb essential physiological pathway of parasites. The cure rate and egg reduction rate tests are commonly used to judge efficacy of anthelmintic in human.

Other test include, egg hatch test, larval development assay and larval arrested morphology assay. Recently, to measure pyrentel sensitivity motility assay and novel assays are developed.

A major class of broad-spectrum anthelmintics is of benzimidazoles (e.g., albendazole, mebendazole and thiabendazole) [1]. The first broad-spectrum anthelmintics thiabendazole was discovered in 1961. Benzimidazoles affect microtubular function of helminth. Mebendazole is usually the drug of choice, and is relatively free of side-effects. Albendazole has superior absorption pattern from blood. Benzimidazoles are widely used to treat worm infections over flukes. The lipophilic albendazole exerts anthelmintic action through transcuticular diffusion by parasitic worms.

Another class of anthelmintics is a nicotinic receptor agonist e.g., levamisole, pyrantel and morantel, causes spastic muscle paralysis. Two drugs of oxindole alkaloid family are used as an anthelmintic. Marcfortine A is active against *C. Elegans* and Paraherquamide and its derivative, 2-deoxy-pa-raherquamide, induces flaccid paralysis in parasitic nematodes.

Paraherquamide interfere with cholinergic transmission. Another broad-spectrum anthelmintic is praziquantel which acts by affecting calcium homeostasis in the parasites, thereby affecting the muscular system resulting in severe paralysis and eventually death.

It is also administered in schistosomiasis. It acts against mature and young fluke parasites. Praziquantel is very safe in humans, and in some cases adverse effects are observed due to the interaction with dead organisms. Pyrentel works on similar mechanism.

Metriphonate particularly used for treating *Schistosoma haematobium* species and piperazine, levamisole, niclosamide for treating roundworm and threadworm infections to quite a large extent. Another piperazine derivative diethylcarbamazine is used to treat filarial infections by increasing the host's immune reaction.

Oxamniquine and metriphonate is drug of choice to treat schistosomiasis. Ivermectin is a semisynthetic derivative of the avermectins prepared from

Streptomyces avermitilis in 1980 introduced by Merck. It is mainly used for treatment of *onchocerciasis* which causes 'river-blindness', and can also be used to treat *Wuchereria bancrofti*, which causes elephantiasis. Ivermectin causes paralysis in parasites through chloride channel opening.

Several other ivermectin analogues like moxidectin, milbemycin oxime, doramectin, selamectin, abamectin and eprinomectin are synthesized further. It is typically not used for STHs because of its relatively low efficacy against hookworms and whipworms.

Another semi-synthetic derivative, emodepside is cyclodepsipeptide. It is produced by fermentation of the fungus (*Mycelia sterilia*). It binds stereo specifically to the receptor and causes muscle paralysis. It shows calcium and potassium dependent mechanism of action. A combination product with praziquantel is available in market for veterinary use.

Combination Therapy

Multiple drug therapy is widely used to treat cancer, bacterial infections, HIV or malaria in human and also in veterinary medicine. Laboratory study showed promising results for combinations of various anthelmintics *in vitro* and *in vivo* against the *T. muris*. In vivo trials showed synergistic properties between, mebendazole-ivermectin, mebendazole-levamisole, albendazole-mebendazole and albendazole plus ivermectin pairs. It is evident that the synergistic combinations comprised atleast one benzimidazoles. Enhanced bioavailability of ivermectin was observed when given with levamisole in healthy volunteers [2].

The mainly studied combinations against *T. muris in vitro* include albendazole-mebendazole, albendazole-levamisole, albendazole-pyrantelpamoate, albendazole-ivermectin, mebendazole-levamisole, mebendazole-pyrantel pamoate, mebendazole-ivermectin, levamisole-pyrantel pamoate, levamisole-ivermectin and pyrantel pamoate-ivermectin [3].

In another study, a significant synergy was reported for tribendimidine or levamisole for Cry proteins from *Bacillus thuringiensis* [7]. Tribendimidine combined with levamisole increased the effectiveness against *Ancylostoma ceylanicum in vitro* and *in vivo* in male Syrian Golden hamsters [8]. Several clinical trials has been conducted with different drug combinations in patients infected with hookworms or *T. trichiura* [4, 9-11], None of the marketed anthelmintics was effective in reducing the larval rates and egg reduction rates at single dose in the treatment of *T. trichiura* [2, 3].

No trichuricidal activity was noted for combination of the mebendazole and levamisole when given to the school-aged children on Pemba island [4].

Similar combination did exhibit notable activity for previously reported combinations of albendazole-ivermectin, mebendazole-ivermectin and albendazole-mebendazole in *T. muris* infected mice.

Another clinical trials showed combination drugs are more effective (with higher cure rate of 46.1%) compared to single drug (albendazole, cure rate 6.0%) and mebendazole (cure rate 11%) in *T. trichiura* infected school children in Uganda [5]. Continuous dosing for 4 to 6 weeks with tetracycline and rifampicin completely flushed out adult filariae.

Other Clinically Active Drugs [6]

Since last six decades piperazine, an OTC drug is mainly used in treating thread worm infections in children. In separate study, antimalarial artemisinin along with their synthetic analogues (trioxane and trioxolane) and mefloquine and its analogue showed helmintic activity. A compound latrophilins is from class of G protein coupled receptors and mainly bind to the neurotoxin and latrotoxin. The mechanism of action is by triggering neurotransmitter release, thereby causing paralysis of muscles. Tribendimidine is a broad spectrum anthelmintics for human use while monepantel in used for therapy in sheep. New anthelmintic drug tribendimidine was recently tested in human. All clinical trials showed very good activity against *Ascaris* and hookworms and also found to be safe. It is L-subtype nAChR agonist and the mechanism of action of tribendimidine is predicted to be same as levamisole and pyrantel [7, 8].

Another intestinal broad spectrum nitazoxanide is a pyruvate ferredoxin oxido reductase inhibitor. It is also used in helmintic therapy depending upon the severity of disease. Till date, anthelmintic therapy is mainly based on very few drugs adapted from veterinary sciences and their combination with some antibiotics. Very few actives or their derivatives are synthesized and studied limitedly. Sanderson B E described in detail the effect of various anthelmintic drugs from category haloxon, metrifonate, crufomate, naphthalophos, phenothiazine, thiabendazole, parbendazole, tetramisole hydrochloride, bephenium hydroxy naphthoate, thenium closylate, pyrvinium pamoate (*Cyanine dyes)*, dithiazanine iodide (*Cyanine dyes)*, methyridine, pyrantel tartrate, piperazine, and diethylcarbamazine on nematodes [9-11].

Tetrahydropyrimidines, imidiathiazoles, macrocylic lactones, piperazine acts mainly on ion channels while benzimidazoles on microtubules. The target is unknown for praziquantel and triclabendazole. Readers can refer cited articles for more details on biomedical mechanism and resistance development of anthelmintics [12-14].

Successful clinical trial of CDRI-81:470, a broad spectrum anthelmintic agent was carried out in 12 healthy human after oral administration at single dose of 375 mg [15] Thiabendazole, mebendazole, levamisole and ivermectin were tested in gullet worm, *Gongylonema pulchrum in vitro* and *in vivo*, separately [16]. A cluster-randomized trial was performed in 1 million pre-school children in India [17]. In another separate open label phase 2 trial, efficacy and safety of mefloquine, artesunate, mefloquine–artesunate, tribendimidine, and praziquantel was evaluated in patients with *Opisthorchis viverrini* [18].

Table 2. Overview of clinical trials in area of helmintic treatments

Title	Sponsor	Completion year	Phase	Identification number	Formulation
A Study to Assess the Efficacy and Safety of Mebendazole for the Treatment of helminth Infections in Pediatric Participants	Janssen Research and Development, LLC	2014	Phase 3	NCT02034162	Single dose of a 500-mg chewable tablet of Mebendazole
Schistosome and Intestinal worm Infections and Malaria Morbidity Among School and Pre-school Children in, Tanzania	DBL -Institute for Health Research and Development	2011	-	NCT00347113	Single dose of Praziquantel 40mg/kg and albendazole 400mg
Empiric Therapy of helminth Co-infection to Reduce HIV-1 Disease Progression (THE or PHE)	University of Washington	2011	-	NCT00507221	Albendazole every 3 months for 24 months 400mg/day X 3 days Praziquantel at enrollment and 12 months: 25mg/kg X 1
Treatment of helminth co-Infection: Short-Term Effects on HIV-1 Progression Markers and Immune Activation	University of Washington	2007	-	NCT00130910	Albendazole (Zentel) 400mg x 3 first dose observed
Monitoring the Efficacy of Anthelmintics for the Treatment of Soil Transmitted helminth P2 (ConWorm)	University Ghent	2012	Phase 4	NCT01379326	Single-dose Mebendazole 500 mg

Table 2. (Continued)

Title	Sponsor	Completion year	Phase	Identification number	Formulation
Effect of Albendazole Dose on Clearance of Filarial worms	National Institute of Allergy and Infectious Diseases (NIAID)	2011	Phase 2	NCT00375583	Standard annual dose diethylcarbamazine 300 mg/Albendazole 400 mg
Optimization of Mass Drug Administration With Existing Drug Regimens for Lymphatic Filariasis and Onchocerciasis (DOLF-Indo)	Washington University School of Medicine	2015	-	NCT01905423	Albendazole (Albenza) 400 mg plus diethylcarbamazine 6 mg/kg once yearly vs twice yearly
Optimization of Mass Drug Administration With Existing Drug Regimens for Lymphatic Filariasis and Onchocerciasis for Liberia (DOLF-LIBERIA)	Washington University School of Medicine	2016		NCT01905436	Annual or semiannual Albendazole (Albenza) 400 mg plus Ivermectin 200 mg (Mectizan or Stromectol)
Antihelminthic Therapy Combined With Antimony in the Treatment of Cutaneous Leishmaniasis	Hospital Universitário Professor Edgard Santos	2009	-	NCT00469495	Anthelmintic meglumine antimony
Effect of Albendazole Dose on Clearance of Filarial worms	National Institute of Allergy and Infectious Diseases (NIAID)	2011	-	NCT00339417	800 mg of albendazole twice a year plus 200 mcg/kg of ivermectin twice a year for 2 years
Comparative Efficacy of Different Mebendazole Polymorphs in the Treatment of Soil-transmitted helminth Infections	University of Kelaniya	2013	Phase 3	NCT01350271	Mebendazole poly-morph A and C 500 mg Mebendazole polymorph C alone

Title	Sponsor	Completion year	Phase	Identification number	Formulation
The Effect of a Deworming Intervention to Improve Early Childhood Growth and Development in Resource-poor Areas	McGill University Health Center	2012	Phase 4	NCT01314937	Single-dose 500 mg mebendazole tablet (Vermox, Nemasole, Pantelmin)
Relative Efficacy of Two Regimens of Ante- helminth Treatment	International Centre for Diarrhoeal Disease Research, Bangladesh	2011		NCT00367627	400 mg of Albendazole in a single dose
Efficacy Albendazole and Levamisole Against STH on Unguja (ALBvLEV)	Natural History Museum, United Kingdoms	2008	Phase 4	NCT00659997	Albendazole Single oral dose of 400mg and levamisole Single oral dose of 2.5mg/kg
A Community Trial for Visceral Leishmaniasis (VL)	International Centre for Diarrhoeal Disease Research, Bangladesh	2012	-	NCT01069198	Albendazole, Iron, Zinc and Vitamin A single oral dose of 200,000 IU Vitamin A at baseline and after six months, 35 mg and 65 oral elemental iron for subject aged <5 and >=5 years respectively everyday for two months starting from enrollment; 10 mg oral zinc for 10 consecutive days each month for 6 months; and a single 400 mg oral dose of albendazole at 3-months' intervals.
A Multinational Trial of the Efficacy of Albendazole Against Soil-transmitted Nematode Infections in Children (WORMCON)	University Ghent	2011	Phase 4	NCT01087099	A single 400 mg dose of albendazole

Several other clinical trials are completed recently for treating various helmintic infection and are listed in Table 2.

A diketopiperazine compound belongs to the category of paraherquamide compounds. Compounds belonging to this class have a common mechanism of action. Marcafortine, paraherquamide A and a semi synthetic derivative of paraherquamide (derquantel) belong to this class. They act as a cholinergic receptor antagonist at the neuromuscular junction of the nematodes thus paralyzing the parasite.

These compounds have selective action against the nematodes due to that sub- minimal dose is required to demonstrate the action. Derquental acts as antagonist at the nicotinic acetylcholine receptors and paralyses the flaccid nematodes.

There are other anthelmintics such as salicylanilides, organophosphates and nitrophenols referred to as narrow spectrum compounds, which have activity against fewer species of parasites such as *Haemonchus contortus* in sheep and/or lack high levels of efficacy against all stages of the parasites.

Helmintic Resistance

Many findings confirms the development of anthelmintic drug or multiple drug resistance in human as well in animals [19, 20]. The proposed reasons could be the occurrence of frequent infections, drug tolerant parasitic infections to the host, genetic mutations in parasites, wrong dose selection (under dose or overdose), dosing frequency, purity of drug (generic or branded product), loss or decrease of target affinity, age related drug distribution issue, drug interaction in combination form, food types that can interference drug action, presence of latent infections and type of dosage form used. Most of the time helmintic infections are overlooked as it leads mainly to subclinical diseases. Simultaneous or rotational use of different drugs should be implemented. Use of drugs having different mechanisms of action might postpone the resistance development to each of the drugs used [21].

Anthelmintics Formulation Developments

Hennessy recommended use of modern drug delivery systems which is formulated wisely until vaccines, biological control and breeding of parasite-resistant animals is available in near future [22]. Formulations strategies can be used to increase the drug availability and anthelmintic effect thereby reducing the dosing frequency and related toxicity effects.

Oral delivery of anthelmintics has been done traditionally in the form of tablet and solution.

Extended release formulations are viable options for human as well as animals e.g., controlled release tablets and capsules. Deeper understanding of anthelmintic pharmacokinetic and dynamic behavior helps science to explore targeting options for multiparticulate formulations.

Solid and Liquid Dosage Forms

Ramaiah M., prepared directly compressed polyherbal tablets. The tablets showed significant anthelmintic activity differences against control and against earthworm *Pheretima posthuma* [23]. In another study, praziquantel syrup versus crushed praziquantel tablets showed similar profile for treatment of intestinal schistosomiasis when tested in the Ugandan preschool children [24]. New anthelmintic compound C.9333 Go./CGP 4540, was successfully evaluated clinically in 65 adult patients with hookworm infection [25]. After tribendimidine approval in China, several clinical studies are carried out against *Ascaris lumbricoides, Trichuris trichiura, Enterobius vermicularis, Opisthorchis viverrini* and *Clonorchis sinensis*, *Strongyloides stercoralis and C. sinensis*. In all cases tribendimidine exhibited high cure rates [26].

Albendazole solid dispersions incorporated into rapid disintegrating tablets which showed superior plasma profile compared to conventional tablet formulation in dog [27]. Metronidazole was incorporated in ethyl cellulose microencapsulates which was further converted into tablet [28]. Colon targeted drug delivery systems of metronidazole was studied [29]. Recently, 10% w/w albendazole pellets were prepared by extrusion/spheronization technique composed of microcrystalline cellulose and lactose. Tween 80 and low molecular weight chitosan were used as additive to enhance dissolution rate of drug. The results indicate an increase in the weight ratio of lactose and chitosan enhanced ABZ dissolution rate [30]. Praziquantel implants containing PEG/poly epsilon caprolactone were manufactured using twin-screw mixing and hot-melt extrusion [31].

Multiparticulate and Nanoformulations

Solid dispersions of mebendazole containing low-substituted hydroxypropylcellulose (L-HPC) was prepared and tested for anthelmintic activity *Trichinella spiralis* in mice. *In vivo* studies showed superior anthelmintic effects up to 3.8 fold for solid dispersions in comparison to recrystallized drug. Enhancement in anthelmintic activity could be because of an increased solubility of mebendazole [32].

Nanosuspensions/nanocrystal technology is widely used to solve solubility related issues. Magnetically tagged metronidazole nanosuspensions were developed and tested against earthworm *Pheretima poi*. Nanosuspension showed promising results at a dose of 10 and 50 mg/ml compared to non-magnetic metronidazole suspension [33]

The solubility of ivermectin was enhanced almost by 450% by surface solid dispersion technique which further constituted to tablet. Fecal egg and tick counting studies in dog confirmed similar performances to that of marketed tablet which ultimately could control endo and ecto parasites infection in animals [34]. Praziquantel was taste masked using solid lipid extrusion which generated small pellets of 0.5 mm [35]. Solumer formulation of albendazole with poloxamer 407 and sodium carboxymethyl cellulose was developed to achieve superior bioavailability and solubility [36]. Praziquantel [37], 1-Nicotinoyl-4-aryl-3-methyl3a,4-dihydropyrazolo pyrazoles [38], flubendazole [39] was incorporated in cyclodextrin to solve solubility issue. Praziquantel solid lipid nanoparticles are also reported [40, 41].

Table 3. List of literature evidences where anthelmintic drugs are incorporated into drug delivery systems like liposomes, nanoemulsions, solid lipid nanoparticles, nanosuspensions, dendrimers and polymeric nanoparticles to treat helmintic infections

Liposome	Metrifonate	Cholinesterase Inhibitors In Liposomes And Their Production And Use US 20080031935 A1
	Niclosamide	Liposomal assembly for therapeutic and/or diagnostic use US7749485 B2
	Praziquantel	Improvement of antischistosomal activity of praziquantel by incorporation into phosphatidylcholine-containing liposomes. Mourão_SC, Costa PI, Salgado HR, Gremião_MP, Int J Pharm. 2005 May 13;295(1-2):157-62.
	Lavimasol	Ascaris suum-vaccination of mice with liposome encapsulated antigen. Lukes S., Vet Parasitol. 1992 Jun; 43(1-2):105-13.
Nanoemulsions	Metrifonate	Silicone vesicles containing actives WO 2005102248 A2

	Praziquantel	Food, Pharmaceutical and Bioengineering Division (232e) Nanoemulsions As Drug Delivery Systems for Poorly Water-Soluble Drugs: Formulation, Transport of Praziquantel Across Caco-2 Cell Monolayers and Cytotoxicity de Campos, V. E. B., Mansur, C. E., Ricci, E. J., da Rocha, S. R., 12 AIChE, 2012 Annual Meeting
	Lavimasol	Study on the Preparation of Compound Ginsenoside and Levamisole Hydrochloride Nanoemulsion and Its Immunologic Enhancement Effect. White paper, April 16, 2012 by China Papers
	Praziquantel	Solid lipid nanoparticle suspension enhanced the therapeutic efficacy of praziquantel against tapeworm S. Xie, B. Pan, B. Shi, Z. Zhang, Xu Zhang, M Wang, and W Zhou, Int J Nanomedicine. 2011; 6: 2367–2374.
Nanosuspensions	Metrifonate	Freeze dried drug nanosuspensions WO 2012140220 A1
Nanosuspensions	Niclosamide	Fabrication of novel niclosamide-suspension using an electrospray system to improve its therapeutic effects in ovarian cancer cells in vitro. Bai, M.Y.; Yang, H.C. Colloids and Surfaces A: Physicochemical and Engineering Aspects vol. 419 February 20, 2013. p. 248-256
Cyclodextrin complex	Metrifonate	Pharmaceutical compositions comprising cyclodextrins US 20020150616 A1
	Niclosamide	Comparison of the aqueous solubilization of practically insoluble niclosamide by polyamidoamine (PAMAM) dendrimers and cyclodextrins. Devarakonda B, Hill RA, Liebenberg W, Brits M, de Villiers MM Int J Pharm. 2005 Nov 4;304(1-2):193-209.

Table 3. (Continued)

	Praziquantel	Improvement of the oral praziquantel anthelmintic effect by cyclodextrin complexation. de Jesus MB, Pinto Lde M, Fraceto LF, Magalhães LA, Zanotti-Magalhães EM, de Paula E., J Drug Target. 2010 Jan;18(1):21-6
	Ivermectin	Preparation of Ivermectin and Terbinafine Cyclodextrin Inclusion Complex L., Zhang, Northwest Univ. of Science and Technology, Master's thesis 2009
Solid dispersions	Metrifonate	Process for producing a solid dispersion of an active ingredient EP 1832281 A1
	Niclosamide	Formulation and evaluation of taste masked niclosamide solid dispersion as chewable tablet, m.Pharm thesis, Rajiv Gandhi university of health sciences Bangalore, India 2013
	Albendazole	Improving the oral bioavailability of albendazole in rabbits by the solid dispersion technique. Kohri_N, Yamayoshi Y, Xin H, Iseki K, Sato N, Todo S, Miyazaki K J Pharm Pharmacol. 1999 Feb;51(2):159-64.
	Praziquantel	Development and Evaluation of Praziquantel Solid Dispersions in Sodium Starch Glycolate, Tropical Journal of Pharmaceutical Research April 2013; 12 (2): 163-168
Solid dispersions	Ivermectin	Solubility enhancement of ivermectn by using solid dispersion technique S. Karande, S Rawat, Y Sharma, M. Kamble, S. Pandya, N. Gandhi, International Journal of Universal Pharmacy and Life Sciences 3(5): 2013 Int J Pharm. 2013 Hydrogen bond replacement--unearthing a novel molecular mechanism of surface solid dispersion for enhanced solubility of a drug for veterinary use. Singh D, Pathak K.
	Praziquantel	Thermoanalytical study of praziquantel-loaded PLGA nanoparticles Rev. Bras. Cienc. Farm. vol.42 no.4 São Paulo Oct./Dec. 2006

		Development of praziquantel-loaded PLGA nanoparticles and evaluation of intestinal permeation by the everted gut sac model. Mainardes RM, Chaud MV, Gremião MP, Evangelista RC, J. Nanosci. Nanotechnol. 2006 Sep-Oct;6(9-10):3057-61.
	Ivermectin	Therapeutic efficacy of poly (lactic-co-glycolic acid) nanoparticles encapsulated ivermectin (nano-ivermectin) against brugian filariasis in experimental rodent model. M. Ali, M. Afzal, M. Verma, S. Bhattacharya, F. J. Ahmad, M. Samim, M. Z. Abidin, A. K. Dinda. (2014) Parasitology Research 113:2, 681-691
Dendrimers	Niclosamide	Comparison of the aqueous solubilization of practically insoluble niclosamide by polyamidoamine (PAMAM) dendrimers and cyclodextrins. Devarakonda, B.; Hill, R. A.; Liebenberg, W.; Brits, M.; de Villiers, M. M. Int. J. Pharm. 2005, 304, 193-209.

Table 3 lists the anthelmintic drugs which are incorporated in novel drug delivery systems like liposomes, solid lipid nanoparticles etc.

Newer drug delivery technologies are making their way to veterinary medicines, thereby solving complicated issues of solubility and bioavailability. The research in this direction is still in an infancy. Hopefully, in coming years collaborations between industry and academia become much stronger to co develop things together. Thereby, changing the face of human anthelmintic medicine.

Anthelmintic Drug Delivery Systems in Veterinary Use

The prevalence of a particular species of nematode affecting the livestock, grazing animals and its treatment depends upon the stage of parasite life cycle.

Few companies that are involved in manufacturing of antihelmintics for veterinary use are Schering plough, Novartis, Pfizer, Merck, Bayer and Boehringer.

Modern alternative techniques for delivery of classic drugs are designed on the principles of diffusion, osmotic processes, to progressive erosion, or through electronic programmed devices. Anthelmintic sustained release systems e.g., for albendazole (Proftril® bolus), morantel tartrate (Paratect®

flex and bolus) ivermectin (Enzec and Alzet, Ivomec SR Bolus), levamisole (Chronominthic bolus), oxfendazol (Synanthic multidose bolus) fenbendazole (Panacur® Bolus). Anthelmintic programmed periodic release systems include Intra Ruminal Pulse Release Electronic Device (IRPRED), Repidose (Auto-worm) and Oxfendazole Pulsed Release Bolus. Such systems offer advantages like less frequent dosing and reduced handling with reduced cost of treatment and herd management. Patent protection for innovator product and thus extension of product life are few other advantages of novel drug delivery systems. However, efficacy, retention, administration methodology and removal of the non –degradable products from the large animals are a few disadvantages. Available drug marketed ruminal drug devices show consistent release profile till pre dermined time. Among them few has sustained drug delivery function. In drug delivery animal, main challenges remain, dissolution of drug in large volume of rumen, degradation of active drugs caused by habitant of microflora in rumen, selection of correct dose and predefining the shelf life of device ensuring the drug release. Mainly, the ruminal delivery devices are based on matrix assisted slower dissolution, erosion and diffusion mechanism. In animals, high density devices or dosage forms are advised. However, the most commonly used dosage forms are liquids, solids, pastes, injectables and some transdermal formulations.

Proftril - Captec

Albendazole was formulated in a novel drug delivery system and the formulation was tested using Ovoscopical tests.

The test revealed that the treated animals remained free of parasite infection for 10-12 weeks after the administration of capsules and that pasture contami-nation with helminths was significantly reduced efficacy of 96.9-99.2% against nematodes *Nematodirus spp., Oesophagostomum spp., Cooperia spp., Tricho-strongylus spp.* and *Trichuris ovis* was obtained. This indicates the efficacy of the developed Proftril captec against nematode infection in animals [42].

Study performed on grazing Corriedale ewes in Kenya to test the effect of sustained release formulation of albendazole. There was significant reduction in fecal egg counts, herbage larval counts and worm burdens present in the gastro intestinal region of the sheep. These formulations were found very effective for upto 95 days since it could sustain the release of the drug for almost 3 months.

Intraruminal Sustained-Release Capsules (IRSRCs)

In a study performed by Munyua et al., the effect on parasitism in grazing Corriedale was assessed. By the use of IRSRC, the fecal egg counts, herbage larval counts and worm burdens of the major gastrointestinal parasites of sheep were significantly reduced. These capsules (dose) exhausted within 3 months of administration, leading to a rise in the count of eggs per gram in the faeces in the treated group towards the end of the study. The study demonstrates a success story of marketed sustained release formulation [43].

Paratect Bolus/Paratec® Flex

Rumen bolus can be prepared by direct compression technique. A mass of solid metals or tablet excipients is compressed directly to form pre dosage form. It can be alternatively manufactured by extrusion using suitable excipients. Paratect is fabricated for sustained delivery of morantel tartarate. The drug is compressed in the ethylene vinyl acetate polymer layer. Furthermore, the sheet is rolled and fixed in this configuration using water soluble film.

Once administered; due to the unique configuration the film is retained at the back of throat of the animal. The water soluble film dissolves; unwinding the role and preventing its regurgitation by the animal. However, due to economic reasons the film had to be withdrawn from the market.

A combination of paratect sustained release bolus and vaccination improved the condition of the calves with reduction in larval output [44]. This type of device can maintain drug levels until 90 days.

Morantel Sustained Release Trilaminate (MSRT) Bolus

The efficacy of MSRT against gastrointestinal nematodes was evaluated in weaner twenty calves. Fecal worm egg counts and herbage larval counts were reduced by 55 to 86% in herbage larval infectivity test. The results indicate the efficacy of the MSRT bolus.

Chronomintic Bolus

A matrix based device made up of polyurethane loaded with levamisole hydrochloride and iron has been designed named as Chronomintic. The device is bored in the centre with capacity to slowly release the anthelmintic drug levamisole. The device releases 2.5 mg of the loaded levamisole drug in first 24 hours and the remaining is released over a period of 90 days.

Rintal 1.9 Pellets Systems

This type of system can be given four times per year at Febantel dose of 7.5 mg/kg. This type of drug delivery devices can release drug at intermittent levels and at time points. Drug release phases are well separated by no drug release phases.

Another system halloway, can monitor drug release by ensuring the degradation of individual compartment of device. On the other hand, Castex system made significant contribution to rumen drug delivery e.g., Rapidose which is mainly based on electrochemical mechanism.

Ruminant Bolus / Ivomec SR Bolus

The Ivomec SR Bolus essentially comprises an osmotic pump that provides a sustained release of ivermectin in the animal at a uniform rate of approximately 12 mg/day for about 135 days [45].

Ivomec SR Bolus proved to be highly effective against economically important gastrointestinal and pulmonary nematodes in cattles such as *Ostertagia ostertagi*, *Trichostrongylus axei, Cooperia punctata, Oesophago-stomum radiatum, Dictyocaulus viviparous*. Systamex with repidose 750 or 1250 is programmed bolus to eradicate the GIT worms in beef animals. Oxfendazole is the drug exerting the ovicidal effect. The bolus contains 5 therapeutic doses which are released for more than 130 days with the first tablet being released by 21 days.

Reticulo-Rumen Device (RRD)

Vandamme et al. has recently investigated the performance of the levamisole hydrochloride tablets encapsulated RRD device assembled using high-density polyethylene elements on grazing calves. They found that RDD could delay and pulse the release of drug as programmed.

Captec® Device

The Captec device is a device that enables the delivery of the drug from a capsule in a controlled release fashion. This device has been specifically design for delivery of anthelmintic agents. The modification has been further introduced by Wunderlich et al. and Rathbone et al. to Captec device. (17, 18) The modern device is more versatile in delivery duration, rate and drug type in comparison to the original Captec device. This device can be loaded with water soluble, lipid soluble to completely insoluble into the rumen of cattle. The release profile can be tailored by alteration in device design from a few days to up to 9 months. Such devices are beneficial as repeated administration of the drug is avoided and thus are animal friendly. Table 4 gathers information on marketed anthelmintic formulation and end user.

A sustained delivery devices or long acting veterinary drug delivery technology are very well welcomed by veterinary sciences. Table 5 list recent patents in anthelmintic drug delivery. However, the success rate is still not as predicted because of lack of basic understanding of these devices, species variations in animal, dose variability and performance differences. Immunization is best method of controlling nematode infection, although the cost is main determining factor.

Table 4. Anthelmintics and their dosage form available in human and veterinary medicine

Drug	Brand Names	Dose /Dosage form	Inteded use	Company
Triclabendazole	Fasinex®	5-15% /oral drench	sheep	Novartis
	Tribenol-50 oral	Triclabendazole 5% oral suspension	calves, cattle, goats and sheep	Interchemie
Piperazine Citrate	Piperin WS	Piperazine citrate 100% watersoluble powder	horses, swine, cattle and poultry	Interchemie
Praziquantal	Biltricide® Tablet	600mg	Human	Bayer
	Cesol®	150 mg tablet	Human	Merck
	Cysticide	500 mg tablet	Human	Merck
	Distoside	600mg tablets	Human	Chandra Bhagat Pharma Ltd
	Droncit®	23 mg	Vet use (Cats)	Bayer
	Drontal®	18.2 mg praziquantel and 72.6 mg pyrantel base as pyrantel pamoate.	Vet use (Cats)	Bayer
	D-worm Chewable tablets		Vet use (For puppies and dogs)	Farnum

Table 4. (Continued)

Drug	Brand Names	Dose /Dosage form	Inteded use	Company
	Milbemax®	2.5mg milbemycin oxime (dose range 0.5-5mg/kg)	Cats and dogs	Novartis
	Propantel	25mg praziquantel	Dogs	jurox
	Profender®	1.8% Emodepside+7.94% Praziquantel/topical solution	Vet use (cats)	Bayer
	Tape worms T	23 mg tablet	Vet use (Cat)	Trade winds
	Zentozide®	600 mg tablets	Human	(Berich) Thailand
Oxaminiquine	Vansil®/ Mansil®	250 mg capsules, syrup 250 mg/5 mL	Human / animal	Pfizer
Albendazole	Valbazen®	Oral Suspension and Paste formulation		Interchemie
	Albenol® 100 oral	10% oral suspension	Goats, sheeps and cattles	Interchemie
	Albenol® 25 oral	2.5% oral suspension	Goats, sheeps and cattles	Interchemie
	Albenol®-2500 Bolus	Bolus for oral administration	Goats, sheeps and cattles	Interchemie
	Albenol® 300 Bolus	Bolus for oral administration	Goats, sheeps and cattles	Interchemie
	Albenol® 600 Bolus	Bolus for oral administration	Goats, sheeps and cattles	Interchemie
	Albenol® 100	10% oral suspension	Cattles	Channelle Animal Health Ltd.
	Albex®	10% oral suspension	Cattles and sheep	Ravensdown
Ricobendazole	Ricomax®	15% Ricobendazole Subcutaneous injection	Cattles	Over cinecia
Flubendazole	Flutelmium®	0.6% premix	Vet use Dogs and cats	Janssen Pharmaceutica N.V
Fenbendazole	Panacur®	3.0 gm or 1.5 gm bolus	sheep, cattle, horses, fish, dogs, cats, rabbits and seals.	Intervet India
	Panacur®	-	horses	Merck
	febenol®- 100 Oral	10% oral suspension	calves, cattle, goats, sheep and swine	Interchemie
Tiabendazole	Mintezol®	25 mg	Human	Merck
Abamectin	Abamectin®	10 g/L injection (endectocide)	Cattles and sheep	Ravensdown
Doramectin	Doramec® L.A.	1g/ 100ml long acting Injectable solution	Cattles	Agrovet Market Animal Health

Drug	Brand Names	Dose /Dosage form	Inteded use	Company
	Dectomax®	1% w/v Doramectin (10mg/mL) Long Acting Injectable Solution	cattle, sheep, swine	Zoetis Australia
	Doraquest L.A.®	1.75% Oral gel	Horses	Agrovet Market animal Health
Ivermectin	Virbac Iverhart®Plus	ivermectin and pyrantal pamoate	Dogs	Virbac
	Tri-Heart® Plus	ivermectin and pyrantal pamoate	Dogs	Intervet
	Stromectol®	3 mg tablets	Human	Merck
	Ivomec® Pour on/ Ivomec® Eprinex® Pour-On	solution	Cattles	Merial Animal Health
	Mectizan®	_	_	Merck
	Intermectin	Ivermectin 1% Injectable solution	calves, cattle, goats, sheep and swine	Interchemie
	Intermectin Duo Paste	Ivermectin 1.55% and praziquantel 7.75% oral paste	Horses and Mares	Interchemie
	Intermectin oral	Ivermectin 0.08% oral drench	calves, sheep and goats	Interchemie
	Intermectin Paste	Ivermectin 1.87% oral paste	Horses	Interchemie
	Intermectin pour on	Ivermectin 0.5% pour-on	veternary use. Contraindicated in lactating animals	Interchemie
	Intermectin Super	Ivermectin 1%, Clorsulon 10% injectable solution	Parentral administration cattles	Interchemie
Ivermectin	Intermectin- 10% drench	Ivermectin 1% Oral Drench	calves, sheep and goats.	Interchemie
	Ivexterm®	_	_	Valeant Pharmaceuticals International
	Scabo® 6	_	_	Delta Pharma Ltd.
	Bovimec®	Ivermectin 1% injectable solution	calves, sheep and goats.	Agrovet Market animal Health
	Boldemec® L.A.	Boldenone undecylenate 2.8 g, ivermectin 1 g long acting injection	calves, sheep and goats.	Agrovet Market animal Health
Noromectin	Noromectin Horse Paste	1.87% Oral paste	Horses	Norbrook
Selamectin	Revolution®	topical solution Available in 8 different strengths	Dogs and cats	Pfizer

Table 4. (Continued)

Drug	Brand Names	Dose /Dosage form	Inteded use	Company
Moxidectin	Cydectin® Pour On	Contains 5 mg moxidectin/mL	dogs, cats, horses, cattle and sheep	Boehringer Ingelheim Vetmedica
Milbemycin	Interceptor®	_	Dogs	Novartis
Milbemycin oxime	Milbemax®	2.5mg milbemycin oxime (dose range 0.5-5mg/kg)	cats and dogs	Novartis
	Milbemax®	25mg praziquantel Chewable tablets	Dogs	Novartis
	Sentinel®	chewable flavored tablet / 0.23 mg/pound (0.5 mg/kg) of milbemycin oxime, 4.55 mg/pound (10 mg/kg) of lufenuron, and 2.28 mg/pound (5 mg/kg) of praziquantel orally/once a month	Dogs	Novartis
Closanthel	Closan-100	10% aqueous solution for parentral administration	Goats, sheeps and cattles	Interchemie
Cloasanthel and Levamisole	Closel-150	Closanthel 5% and Levamisole HCl 10% injectable suspension	Goats, sheeps and cattles	Interchemie
Nitroxinil	Fluconix- 340	Nitroxinil 345 Injectable solution	cattle and sheep	Interchemie
Levamisole	Interzan Gold Oral	Levamisole HCl 3%, Oxyclozanide 6% oral suspension	cattle, calves, sheep and goats	Interchemie
	Interzan® Oral	Levamisole HCl 1.5%, Oxyclozanide 3% oral suspension	cattle, calves, sheep and goats	Interchemie
	Leva®-100	Levamisole 10% Injectable solution	Calves, cattle, goats, sheep and swine	Interchemie
Levamisole	Leva®-200 Oral	Levamisole HCl 20% oral solution	cattle, calves, sheep, goats, poultry and swine	Interchemie
	Leva®-200 WS	Levamisole HCl 20% powder for oral solution	cattle, calves, sheep, goats, poultry and swine	Interchemie

The outcomes of research done until now shows successful use of sustained/ controlled/ bolus drug delivery systems in animals. New application devices and novel excipients are enhancing their effectiveness day by day.

Herbal Remedies in Human and Veterinary Medicine

Anthelmintics are also known as vermifuges or vermicides. Natural anthelmintic includes medicinal active from tobacco, walnut, wormwood, clove, garlic, malefern, pineapple, diatomaceous earth, soya and other legumes. There have been considerable efforts being taken up in identifying the active ingredients present in indigenous plants possessing anthelmintic activity but there are few plants that have lived up to their expectations when tested rigorously. Tobacco, pyrethrum, rotenone and nicotine agonist acts as acetyl choline agonist and can be used at sub-toxic doses. In fact, nicotine and pyrethrum has provided the template for designing of nicotine agonist class compounds (20a). Copper sulphate act as irritating agent to the nematodes and dislodges them from the host site causing their excretion along with the mucus of the bowels. However substantial toxicity and low efficacy are the associated problems with copper sulphate. Compounds like diatomaceous earth and herbs like pumpkin seeds, garlic and worm wood have been tested for their effect against parasites. Getachew et al. studied the anthelmintic activity of methanol extracts of plants such as leaves of *Myrsine Africana, Rhus glabrous, Jasminum abysinicum, Rhus vulgaris, Acokanthera schimperi* and aerial parts of *Foenicum vulgare* from various part of Africa on nematode parasite, *Heamonchus contortus* was assessed using the egg hatch test and larval Development test. The methanolic and aqueous extracts of *F. vulgare* were as effective as albendazole in inhibiting the egg hatching (IC50 for egg hatching of *F. Vulgare* and Albendazole was 0.25 mg/ ml).

The extracts of other compounds were effective at high concentrations in inhibiting the egg hatching with no statistical difference in inhibition of egg hatching between the aqueous and alcoholic extract. For the larval inhibition, alcoholic extract of *R. glabrous* (97.7%) demonstrated good activity while the least effective plant was aqueous extract of *R. vulgaris* (10%) at the maximum tested concentration. Dose dependent inhibition of larval development was noted, with statistical difference in the counterparts extracts [46].

Some of the earliest known medicinal anthelmintic plants include papaya (*Carica papaya*), figs (*Ficus spp.*) and pineapple (*Ananas comosus*) are known to clear the nematodes and clear intestinal worms, *Trichuris trichiura* in humans. The cysteine proteinases enzymes from these plants responsible for potential activity include papain, chymopapain, caricain, glycyl endopeptidase ficin, ficain ananain, fruit bromelain, stem bromelain, Comosain Actinidain

Asclepain mucunain. Honey, warm water and vinegar together also acts as a good vermifuges. The essential oils anethole and thymol from the plants were found to be exhibit the action against nematodes. Although, there is a lot of literature available on herbal agents to be used as anthelmintics, however very limited data on toxicology and efficacy is available. Further, the number of test animals is very small and validation of such studies is question mark. Effective methodology to investigate the inhibition of motility, larvacidal activity and egg killing activity is urgently required. On a commercial ground; variability in the concentration of active principles in relation to how the plants were grown, climate, soil quality, site, and season of the year play important role.

Table 5. Patents on anthelmintic for veterinary use

Patent	Year	Applicant	Abstract	Drug (if any)
WO2013043064 A1	2013	Alleva Animal Health Limited	Veterinary anthelmintic delivery system	Macrocyclic lactone anthelmintics and Levamisole
US 7667095 B2	2010	Divergence, Inc.	Transgenic plants having anthelmintic activity and methods of producing them	DNA
US 7563773 B2	2009	Merial Limited	Anthelmintic oral homogeneous veterinary pastes	Praziquantel and/or pyrantel, and at least one marcrolide anthelmintic
EP 2 170 321 B1	2009	Pfizer Animal Health	Anthelmintic combination	2-Desoxoparaherqua mide and abamectin
US 20080249153	2008	Razzak, Majid Hameed Abdul	Anthelmintic formulations	Triclabendazole

Future Challenges

The constant reports related to the failure of anthelmintic devices and drugs due to the resistance created in grazing animals demonstrates the challenges posed by a successful anthelmintic therapy in veterinary practice. The two ways to control the parasitic infection is use of anthelmintics in veterinary practice as adjuncts to the control of parasitic disease, and as curative agents when prophylaxis has not been practiced or when it has failed. Limitations such as effect at only few stages of parasite, failure in treating all stages of parasites and ineffective removal of parasites form the body represents an incomplete answer to the control of helminths. Such limitations transform an immature form of parasite to a more important pathogen in the form of sexually mature adult aggregating the problem in animals. Thus, combination of drugs to cure the pathogenic condition should be tried rather than depending on just one drug for parasitic infection. Prophylactic or preventive measures are better than curative measures. Chances of acquisition of the nematode by the grazing host of the infective stages of the parasite through improvements in animal husbandry and grassland management can be managed. Since the pasture rather than the parasite themselves are the main host for such parasitic infections. Periodical dosing of animals constantly exposed to infection is one method by which this may be achieved. Further new agents that have not yet shown any resistance in animals should be tried for treatment purpose. Such agents have novel mechanism of action that takes benefit of normal physiology of the nematode and parasites; thus infecting only the parasites and not the host. Combination of synthetic compounds with herbal agents is one of the best alternatives as prophylactic measure to protect the animals.

A few new alternatives and measures are being addressed and studied as a part of research investigations as indicated in the patents filed on anthelmintics for veterinary use. Readers can refer other chapters in this book for detail information on helminthiasis and vaccines. To dip dive in vaccine and to get full understand-ding on it refer [47-51].

Conclusion

It is difficult to maintain helmintic parasites in continuous culture which makes it unsuitable for inclusion in high throughput screening test. However, it can be used for screening selective chemical libraries. Tradition anthel-minths are still finding their way to be a modern pharma product thereby reducing these infections at mass scale. Many new anthelmintics are reported to be active against wide range of helminthes. These active if delivered in most suitable pharmaceutical form could help in reduction of anthelmintic cases. The traditional knowledge is still hidden in many parts of world. Strong collaboration with different science streams, better in vitro identification and genetic testing methods, full understanding of anthelmintic pharmacodynamic, resistance mechanisms and finding suitable helmintic model to study activity of new chemical entities of anthelmintic drugs are the targets for future successful anthelmintic therapy.

References

[1] Horton, J., Albendazole: a review of anthelmintic efficacy and safety in humans. *Parasitology*, 2000. 121 Suppl.: p. S113-32.

[2] Awadzi K, E. G., Duke, B. O., Opoku, N. O., Attah, S. K., Addy, E. T., Ardrey, A. E., The co-administration of ivermectin and albendazole-safety, pharmacokinetics and efficacy against Onchocerca volvulus. *Ann. Trop. Med. Parasitol.* 2003. 97: p. 165-178.

[3] Keiser, J., et al., Effect of combinations of marketed human anthelmintic drugs against Trichuris muris in vitro and in vivo. *Parasites and vectors*, 2012. 5: p. 292.

[4] Albonico, M., et al., Efficacy of mebendazole and levamisole alone or in combination against intestinal nematode infections after repeated targeted mebendazole treatment in Zanzibar. *Bulletin of the World Health Organization*, 2003. 81(5): p. 343-52.

[5] Namwanje, H., N. B. Kabatereine and A. Olsen, Efficacy of single and double doses of albendazole and mebendazole alone and in combination in the treatment of Trichuris trichiura in school-age children in Uganda. *Transactions of the Royal Society of Tropical Medicine and Hygiene*, 2011. 105(10): p. 586-90.

[6] Lanusse, C., L. Alvarez and A. Lifschitz, Pharmacological knowledge and sustainable anthelmintic therapy in ruminants. *Veterinary Parasitology*, 2013.

[7] Hu, Y. and Xiao, S.-H., The New Anthelmintic Tribendimidine is an L-type (Levamisole and Pyrantel) Nicotinic Acetylcholine Receptor Agonist. *PLoS Negl. Trop. Dis.*, 2009. 3(8): p. e499.

[8] Hu Y, E. B., Yiu, Y. Y., Miller, M. M., Urban, J. F., et al., n Extensive Comparison of the Effect of Anthelmintic Classes on Diverse Nematodes. *PLoS ONE*, 2013. 8(7): p. e70702.

[9] Sanderson, B. E., The effects of anthelmintics on nematode metabolism. *Comparative and General Pharmacology*, 1970. 1(2): p. 135-51.

[10] Martin, R. J., Modes of action of anthelmintic drugs. *Veterinary Journal*, 1997. 154(1): p. 11-34.

[11] Frayha, G. J., et al., The mechanisms of action of antiprotozoal and anthelmintic drugs in man. *General Pharmacology*, 1997. 28(2): p. 273-99.

[12] Kohler, P., The biochemical basis of anthelmintic action and resistance. *International Journal for Parasitology*, 2001. 31(4): p. 336-45.

[13] Geary, T. G., et al., Unresolved issues in anthelmintic pharmacology for helminthiases of humans. *International Journal for Parasitology*, 2010. 40(1): p. 1-13.

[14] Sangster, N. C., Anthelmintic resistance: past, present and future. *International Journal for Parasitology*, 1999. 29(1): p. 115-24; discussion 137-8.

[15] Nagaraja, N. V., et al., Preliminary observations on the pharmacokinetics of CDRI compound 81/470 in calves. *Veterinary Research Communications,* 1998. 22(1): p. 67-72.

[16] Kudo, N., et al., Efficacy of thiabendazole, mebendazole, levamisole and ivermectin against gullet worm, Gongylonema pulchrum: in vitro and in vivo studies. *Veterinary Parasitology*, 2008. 151(1): p. 46-52.

[17] Awasthi, S., et al., Population deworming every 6 months with albendazole in 1 million pre-school children in North India: DEVTA, a cluster-randomised trial. *Lancet*, 2013. 381(9876): p. 1478-86.

[18] Soukhathammavong, P., et al., Efficacy and safety of mefloquine, artesunate, mefloquine-artesunate, tribendimidine, and praziquantel in patients with Opisthorchis viverrini: a randomised, exploratory, open-label, phase 2 trial. *The Lancet infectious diseases*, 2011. 11(2): p. 110-8.

[19] Jozef Vercruysse a, Marco Albonico b, Jerzy M. Behnke c, Andrew C. Kotze d, Roger K. Prichard e, and A.M.g. James S. McCarthy f, Bruno Levecke a, Is anthelmintic resistance a concern for the control of human soil-transmitted helminths? *International Journal for Parasitology: Drugs and Drug Resistance*, 2011(1): p. 14-27.

[20] Anne Lespine, et al., P-glycoproteins and other multidrug resistance transporters in the pharmacology of anthelmintics: Prospects for reversing transport-dependent anthelmintic resistance. *International Journal for Parasitology: Drugs and Drug Resistance*, 2012(2): p. 58-75.

[21] Geerts, S. and B. Gryseels, Drug resistance in human helminths: current situation and lessons from livestock. *Clinical Microbiology Reviews*, 2000. 13(2): p. 207-22.

[22] Hennessy, D. R., Modifying the formulation or delivery mechanism to increase the activity of anthelmintic compounds. *Veterinary Parasitology,* 1997. 72(3-4): p. 367-82; discussion 382-90.
[23] Ramaiaha, M., G. Chakravathib and K. Yasaswinia, In vitro biological standardization, formulation and evaluation of directly compressed polyherbal anthelmintic tablets. *Pharmacognosy Journal*, 2013. 5(3): p. 130-134.
[24] Navaratnam, A. M., et al., Efficacy of praziquantel syrup versus crushed praziquantel tablets in the treatment of intestinal schistosomiasis in Ugandan preschool children, with observation on compliance and safety. *Transactions of the Royal Society of Tropical Medicine and Hygiene*, 2012. 106(7): p. 400-7.
[25] Vakil, B. J., N. J. Dalal and P. N. Shah, Clinical evaluation of a new anthelmintic — C.9333 Go./CGP 4540 in human hookworm infection. *Tropical Medicine and Hygiene*, 1977. 71(3): p. 247-250.
[26] Xiao, S. H., et al., Advances with the Chinese anthelminthic drug tribendimidine in clinical trials and laboratory investigations. *Acta Tropica*, 2013. 126(2): p. 115-26.
[27] Castro, S. G., et al., Comparative plasma exposure of albendazole after administration of rapidly disintegrating tablets in dogs. *Bio. Med. research international*, 2013. 2013: p. 920305.
[28] Ahmad, M., et al., Pharmacokinetic modelling of microencapsulated metronidazole. *Yao xue xue bao = Acta pharmaceutica Sinica*, 2009. 44 (6): p. 674-9.
[29] Kotla Niranjan*, A. S., Jagadish Muthyala, Pandya Pinakin, Effect of Guar Gum and Xanthan Gum Compression Coating on Release Studies of Metronidazole in Human Fecal Media for Colon Targeted Drug Delivery Systems. *Asian Journal of Pharmaceutical and Clinical Research,* 2013. 6(2): p. 315-318.
[30] Ibrahima, M. A. and F. K. Al-Anazia, Enhancement of the dissolution of albendazole from pellets using MTR technique, *Saudi Pharmaceutical Journal,* 2013. 21(2): p. 215-223.
[31] Cheng, L., L. Lei and S. Guo, In vitro and in vivo evaluation of praziquantel loaded implants based on PEG/PCL blends. *International Journal of Pharmaceutics,* 2010. 387(1-2): p. 129-38.
[32] Garcia-Rodriguez, J. J., et al., Changed crystallinity of mebendazole solid dispersion: improved anthelmintic activity. *International Journal of Pharmaceutics,* 2011. 403(1-2): p. 23-8.

[33] Subbiah Lathaa, et al., Formulation development and evaluation of metronidazole magnetic nanosuspension as a magnetic-targeted and polymeric-controlled drug delivery system. *Journal of Magnetism and Magnetic Materials,* 2009. 321(10): p. 1580-1585.

[34] Singh, D. and K. Pathak, Hydrogen bond replacement--unearthing a novel molecular mechanism of surface solid dispersion for enhanced solubility of a drug for veterinary use. *International Journal of Pharmaceutics,* 2013. 441(1-2): p. 99-110.

[35] Witzleb, R., et al., Solid lipid extrusion with small die diameters--electrostatic charging, taste masking and continuous production. *European journal of pharmaceutics and biopharmaceutics: official journal of Arbeitsgemeinschaft fur Pharmazeutische Verfahrenstechnik* e.V, 2011. 77(1): p. 170-7.

[36] Galia Temtsin Krayz, P. M. A., PhD; Anna Berman, MSc; Amir Zalcenstein, PhD, MBA; and and P. Irene Jaffe, Oral DeliveryWith Novel Solid Dispersions: Stable Self-Assembled Formulations of Lipophilic Drugs With Improved Bioperformance. *Drug Delivery Technology* July/August 2009 Vol. 9 No. 7, 2013: p. 32-46.

[37] De Jesus, M. B., et al., Improvement of the oral praziquantel anthelmintic effect by cyclodextrin complexation. *Journal of Drug Targeting,* 2010. 18(1): p. 21-6.

[38] Singh, S. P.a.D. L., Study of anthelmintic properties of 1-Nicotinoyl-4-aryl-3-methyl 3a,4-dihydropyrazolo[3,4c] pyrazoles and their inclusion complexes with β-cyclodextrin. *Journal of Chemical and Pharmaceutical Research,* 2013. 5(5): p. 374-381.

[39] Laura Ceballos1, Laura Moreno1,2, Juan J Torrado2,3, Carlos Lanusse 1, 2 and Luis Alvarez 1,2, Exploring flubendazole formulations for use in sheep. Pharmacokinetic evaluation of a cyclodextrin-based solution. *BMC Veterinary Research* 2012. 8: p. 71.

[40] Xie, S., et al., Formulation, characterization and pharmacokinetics of praziquantel-loaded hydrogenated castor oil solid lipid nanoparticles. *Nanomedicine*, 2010. 5(5): p. 693-701.

[41] Xie, S., et al., Solid lipid nanoparticle suspension enhanced the therapeutic efficacy of praziquantel against tapeworm. *International Journal of Nanomedicine*, 2011. 6: p. 2367-74.

[42] Corba, J., et al., Effect of bolus administration of albendazole into the rumen on gastrointestinal nematodes and the Dicrocoelium dendriticum trematode in sheep. *Vet. Med.* (Praha.), 1994. 39(6): p. 297-304.

[43] Munyua, W. K., et al., The effects of a controlled-release albendazole capsule (Profitril-Captec) on parasitism in grazing Corriedale ewes in the Nyandarua district of Kenya. *Veterinary Research Communications*, 1997. 21(2): p. 85-99.

[44] Hendriks, J., et al., he prophylactic effect of a morantel sustained release bolus (Paratect) on lungworm infections in vaccinated and non-vaccinated calves. *Tijdschrift voor diergeneeskunde*, 1983. 108(3): p. 90-96.

[45] Rathborne, M. J., Delivering drugs to farmed animals using controlled release science and technology. *IeJSME*, 2012. 6: p. S118-128.

[46] Getachew, S., et al., In vitro Evaluation of Anthelmintic Activities of Crude Extracts of Selected Medicinal Plants Against Haemonchus Contortus in Alemgena Wereda, Ethiopia. *Acta Parasitologica Globalis*, 2012. 3(2): p. 20-27.

[47] Pearson, M. S., N. Ranjit and A. Loukas, Blunting the knife: development of vaccines targeting digestive proteases of blood-feeding helminth parasites. *Biological Chemistry*, 2010. 391(8): p. 901-11.

[48] Geldhof, P., et al., Recombinant expression systems: the obstacle to helminth vaccines? *Trends in parasitology*, 2007. 23(11): p. 527-32.

[49] Smith, W. D. and D. S. Zarlenga, Developments and hurdles in generating vaccines for controlling helminth parasites of grazing ruminants. *Veterinary Parasitology*, 2006. 139(4): p. 347-59.

[50] Meeusen, E. N. and J. F. Maddox, Progress and expectations for helminth vaccines. *Advances in Veterinary Medicine*, 1999. 41: p. 241-56.

[51] McManus, D. P., Helminth vaccines. *Biotechnology*, 1992. 20: p. 99-128.

In: Anthelmintics
Editor: William Quick
ISBN: 978-1-63117-714-9

Chapter 3

The Genetic Basis of Anthelminthic Drug Resistance in *Trichostrongylid* Nematodes

***Rafael R. Assis*[1], *Livia L. Santos*[2], *Eduardo Bastianetto*[3], *Denise A. A de Oliveira*[2] *and Bruno S. A. F. Brasil*[4*]**
[1]Laboratório de Laboratório de Parasitologia Celular e Molecular, Fiocruz, MG, Brazil
[2]Laboratório de Genética Animal
[3]Laboratório de Parasitologia, Escola de Veterinária, Universidade Federal de Minas Gerais, Brazil
[4]Embrapa Agroenergia, Brasília, DF, Brazil

Abstract

Trichostrongylid nematodes are important parasites of domestic ruminants and are responsible for significant economic losses in tropical and temperate regions. After years of widespread use of anthelminthic drugs, the increasing prevalence of resistant nematodes now threatens the production of livestock in several parts of the world.

The continued drug use did not eradicate the parasites, mainly because the majority of the nematode populations are in *refugia* (e.g., eggs and larvae in the pasture or inside untreated asymptomatic animals), therefore not submitted to drug selection. Consequently, the genetic pool present in the populations in *refugia* continuously supply genetic variability, sometimes in the form of drug resistance conferring mutations, which eventually became fixed. The situation is further complicated by the high gene flow among parasite populations and their high mutation rates.

Indeed there are several reports describing that resistance can originate through different ways such as animal movement among farms and novel/recurrent mutations. Therefore considerable efforts are being made to develop tests for the diagnosis of anthelminthic resistance that would allow the establishment of rational and sustainable programs for the control of nematode populations in livestock. In this context, molecular tests based on the analysis of resistance-associated target gene polymorphisms become attractive since they present high sensitivity and can deliver precise results in shorter periods of time than traditional techniques.

A major drawback for the development of molecular tests, though, is the poor knowledge about the genetic mutations associated with the resistant phenotypes for most drug classes. In here, it is described the current knowledge about the molecular basis of anthelminthic drug resistance and the prevalence of resistance in different *Trichostrongylid* species. Anthelminthic drug resistance rise and spread is also discussed in the context of nematode population genetics dynamics.

Introduction

Antiparasitic drugs are important tools widely used to maintain animal welfare. As parasites impart a great impact on animal health, these drugs are often essential for the expression of the full genetic potential of production. However, despite the initial success, after years of massive use of anthelminthic drugs (ATH), the increase in prevalence of resistant nematodes became a major problem (Prichard, 2001). Therefore, during the last decade alternative models for sustainable prevention and control of parasites has become a growing need. These programs aim on reducing the impact of the parasite infection as well as reducing the frequency of treatments, therefore, minimizing the selective pressure imposed upon parasite's populations (Sutherland and Leathwick, 2011).

These strategies, however, need a rational use of the right drugs in the correct frequency and, therefore, require a solid base on the biology of the parasites together with efficient diagnostic tools to identify the correct species, resistant variants and the availability of high efficiency drugs. Additionally, other aspects of the helminthic infections must be taken into consideration: Most of the natural infections occur with multiple species that coexist inside the same host; Different host species might live in the same environment; ATH drugs might have different efficiency in different parasite species. Additionally, the high biotic potential, short period between population generations and broad host spectrum observed on the main trichostrongylid species reflect on a rapid increase on the prevalence of mutiresistant parasites.

Anti-Helminthic Resistance in *Trichostrongylidae*

To date, ATH resistance has been described worldwide, mainly in warm temperate or tropical regions of the world (Waller and Prichard, 1986). The rate of emergence of resistance to ATH vary in intensity, mainly in accordance with the prevailing climate, parasite species and ATH treatment regimens adopted (Jabbar et al., 2006). The majority of the anthelmintic resistance cases reported in livestock involves infections with worms from the *Trichostrongylidae* family (Sutherland and Leathwick, 2011; Jackson and Coop, 2000), mostly from the genus *Haemonchus*, *Trichostrongylus*, *Cooperia* and *Teladorsagia* (Table 1). ATH resistance against all the three broad-spectrum drug families (Benzimidazoles; Imidazothiazoles and Tetrahydropyrimidines; Macrocyclic Lactones) has been recorded in many countries (Table 1) (Prichard et al., 1980; Coles, 1986; Waller, 1987; Prichard, 1990). Resistance has been recorded also in drugs with a narrower spectrum of activity such as the salicylanilides (Jeannin et al., 1990; Scott and Armour, 1991). In the early days of ATH resistance in ruminants, resistance was usually detected as a single parasite species resistant to a single class of anthelmintic. Over time, as resistance became more prevalent, more cases which involved more than one species and/or >1 class of anthelmintic appeared. This might be expected given the continued selection of resistance conferring mutations by the use of multiple types of drugs simultaneously or intercalated in a short period of time.

Recent studies continue to report significant prevalence levels of resistance to Benzimidazoles (BZ) reported in Australia (Love, 2007), Europe (Papadopoulos, 2008), New Zealand (Waghorn et al., 2006; Leathwick et al., 2000), United States (Howell et al., 2008) and Brazil (Sczesny-Moraes et al.,2010; daCruz et al., 2010; Nunes et al., 2013) - mainly for the genera

Haemonchus, Trichostrongylus, Teladorsagia and *Ostertagia*. The majority of the cases involve infection of small ruminants (Table 1). Nonetheless, cases of BZ resistance in cattle were reported in Argentina (Anziani et al., 2004; Suarez and Cristel, 2007), Brazil (Soutello et al., 2007), New Zealand (Jackson et al., 1987; Mc Kenna, 1991; Hosking et al., 1996; Waghorn et al., 2006) and United States (Gasbarre et al., 2009a; Gasbarre et al., 2009b) for the genera *Cooperia, Haemonchus, Ostertagia* and *Trichostrongylus* (Sutherland and Leathwick, 2011). Resistance to Levamizol (LEV), an Imidazothiazoles /Tetrahydro pyrimidines (IT) class drug, in sheep and goat nematodes was also described in these cited regions mainly for the genera *Haemonchus, Trichostrongylus* and *Teladorsagia* (Table 1), but is less prevalent than BZ resistance. For example, in USA, LEV continues to be the most effective drug on most farms, but resistance to this drug is being diagnosed with increased frequency (Kaplan, 2012). In cattle, there are reports of resistance to LEV in Brazil (Soutello et al., 2007) and New Zealand (Waghorn et al., 2006).

The very first case of ivermectin (IVM) resistance was reported in South Africa (Van Wyk et al., 1987), and it has been suggested that this country has particularly severe problems with anthelmintic resistance (Van Wyk et al., 1999). Resistance to macrocyclic lactones (ML) in goat and sheep flocks has also been detected in Australia (Besier and Love, 2003), Brazil (da Cruz et al., 2010), USA (Howell et al., 2008), New Zealand (Waghorn et al., 2006; Leathwick et al., 2000), Europe (Sargison et al., 2010; Schnyder et al. 2005; Artho et al.,2007) – mainly for *Haemonchus spp.*(Table 1). Over the past decade an increasing prevalence of ML resistance in gastrointestinal nematodes of cattle worldwide have been reported. Most involve *Haemonchus, Ostertagia* and *Cooperia* found in Argentina (Anziani et al., 2004; Fiel et al., 2001; Suarez and Cristel, 2007), Australia (Lyndal-Murphy et al., 2009), Brazil (Borges et al., 2005; Soutello et al., 2007; Borges et al., 2008; Condi et al., 2009), Europe (Stafford and Coles, 1999; Demeler et al., 2009), New Zealand (Loveridge et al., 2003; Waghorn et al., 2006; Mason and Mc Kay, 2006) and USA (Gasbarre et al., 2009a; Gasbarre et al., 2009b; Edmonds et al., 2010) (Table 1).

Table 1. ATH drug resistance prevalence in trichostrongylids worldwide

Species	Preferable Host	Oviposition Rate	Pre-Patent Period (Days)	ATH	Region
Haemonchus spp.	Ruminants	5.000-10.000		ML	Argentina, Brazil
				BZ, IT	Argentina, Brazil, Australia
H. placei	Cattle		23-28	ML	Argentina, Brazil, USA
				BZ	Argentina, USA, France
H. contortus	Sheeps and Goats		18-21	ML	South America, USA, India, Kenya, Malaysia, New Zealand, South Africa, UK
				BZ	South America, Australia, USA, Belgium, France, Germany, India, Kenya, Malaysia, New Zealand, Pakistan, South Africa, United Kingdom, Zimbabwe
				IT	South America, Australia, France, India, Kenya, Malaysia, New Zealand, Zimbabwe
Cooperia spp.	Ruminants	100-2000		ML	Argentina, Australia, USA, New Zealand, United Kingdom, India
				BZ	Argentina, USA, New Zealand
				IT	Argentina
C. oncophora	Cattle		12-15	ML	Argentina, Belgium, Sweden, Germany , New Zealand
				BZ	New Zealand
C. punctata	Cattle		11-19	ML	Brazil
C. pectinata	Cattle		12-15	ML	Brazil
Ostertagia spp.	Ruminants	200-300		ML	Argentina, Netherlands, Uruguay
				BZ	Argentina, Australia, Denmark, France, New Zealand, Netherlands, Uruguay

Table 1. (Continued)

Species	Preferable Host	Oviposition Rate	Pre-Patent Period (Days)	ATH	Region
O. ostertagi	Cattle		18-25	IT	Argentina, Australia, France, Netherlands, Uruguay
				ML	Argentina, Denmark, Germany, Belgium, Sweden, USA
				BZ	Argentina, New Zealand
				IT	Belgium, Denmark
Trichostrongylus spp.	Mammals and Birds	100-200		BZ	Argentina, Australia, France, New Zealand, Kenya, Netherlands
				IT	Argentina, Australia, France, Kenya
				ML	Argentina, New Zealand
T. axei	Ruminants		24-25	BZ	Australia
T. longispicularis	Sheep and Cattle		15-23	ML	New Zealand
T. colubriformis	Sheep, Cattle and Goats		15-23	BZ, IT	Australia, Malaysia
				ML	Malaysia

BZ: Benzimidazoles; ML: Macrocyclic Lactones; IT: Imidazothiazoles and Tetrahydropyrimidines.

Note: This list presents does not intend to be an exhaustive list of all the cases of ATH resistance reported to date.

Molecular Basis of Anti-Helminthic Resistance in *Trichoestrongylidae*

The mechanisms by which, drug resistance arise in parasites are complex and are related to multiple factors such as parasite genetics, hosts species and management strategies. The complexity of this issue, have made very difficult to understand and also, to develop strategies to prevent and control resistance. For this reason, there are still many questions still unanswered, specially, concerning the molecular and genetic aspects of resistance. However, much progress has been made and it is described in here the current knowledge of the molecular mechanisms by which drug resistance arise in parasite trichostrongylid nematodes.

As for many other model organisms such as bacteria and yeast, drug resistance in trichoestrongylid nematodes can be classified in a few different basic mechanisms: One mechanism can be the up-regulation of the cellular efflux apparatus, for example, ATP-Binding Cassette (ABC) transporters genes; A second mechanism would involve the alteration in drug targets, usually a result of single nucleotide polymorphisms (SNPs) that make the target immune to drug binding - such as the case for Benzimidazole resistance; A third type of strategy might be the reduction of the availability of the drug target as consequence of gene/protein expression down regulation; And a forth mechanism would involve increased drug metabolism. However, this later mechanism does not seem to be as important as the other aforementioned mechanisms in trichoestrongylids, since ATH drugs tend to form long lasting stable binding to its targets.

Benzimidazoles

To date, the understanding of resistance to BZ and its mode of action is the most advanced (Table 2). Although there were initially compelling evidence to a distinct mode of action (McCracken and Stillwell, 1991), it was proposed that BZ exerts its activity by binding to the cytoskeletal protein tubulin. This causes an inhibition of the formation of microtubules and blocks normal function of the cell (Davidse and Flach, 1977; Lacey and Watson, 1985; Lacey and Prichard, 1986). Due to its success in the control of nematode parasites, BZs were widely used and resistance has become more and more frequent. This binding to tubulin was later shown to be inversely proportional to known resistant isolates in *Haemonchus contortus* (Lacey et al., 1987; Lubega and Prichard, 1991a; b). This was further investigated and it was shown that the majority of BZ- susceptible field isolates display multiple alleles on a single beta-tubulin locus and that most of these alleles were not present in resistant isolates (Roos et al., 1990; Kwa et al., 1993). Later, RFLP data showed that BZ resistance was linked to a similar profile of the beta-tubulin locus both in *Trichostrongylus colubriformis* and *H. contortus*, which supported the hypothesis that beta-tubulin is the major target of selection by BZ (Grant et al., 1996).

In *H. contortus*, two beta-tubulin isotypes were first identified, *beta-tubulin 1* and *2* (Geary et al., 1992; Kwa et al., 1993). Close related orthologs were also identified in *Cooperia oncophora; Teladorsagia circumcincta and Trichostrongylus colubriformis* (Njue and Prichard, 2003). Although, recently, using bioinformatics, two other isotypes were identified in *H. contortus* (Saunders et al., 2013), these are expressed in low quantities and were shown to be orthologs to *C. elegans Cel-mec-7* and *Cel-tbb-4* genes. Additionally, in vitro studies, showed that a selection of a *beta-tubulin 1* isotype allele was directly related to BZ resistance (Roos et al., 1990; Kwa et al., 1993). Accordingly, sequence analysis of this allele revealed the substitution of a Phenylalanine to a Tyrosine at the codon 200 that confers the BZ resistant phenotype due to a single nucleotide mutation (Geary et al., 1991; Kwa et al., 1993). This was later confirmed by functional analysis of *H. contortus* beta-tubulin heterologous expressed into *C. elegans* (Kwa et al., 1995).

Later, another SNP was described to confer BZ resistance in trichostrongylid nematodes. A mutation at the codon 167 of the *beta-tubulin 1* from *T. circumcincta* and *H. contortus* was found in field isolates (Silvestre et al., 2001). This mutation also causes substitution of a Phenylalanine to a Tyrosine, but it's much rarer than F200Y mutation and the impact on the worm fitness is not well understood. More recently, another SNP candidate was characterized on *beta-tubulin 1* gene that is capable of conferring BZ resistance, a glutamate to alanine substitution at the codon 198, observed in benomyl (a Benzimidazole drug) resistant isolates of *Monilinia fructicola* a pathogenic fungi. This mutation was observed in BZ resistant field isolates and interestingly was not found together with the well known F200Y mutation, which suggests that the double mutation may render the worm development unviable (Ghisi et al., 2007). This mutation was later confirmed by *in vitro* selection of BZ resistant *H. contortus* (Rufener et al., 2009).

Macrocyclic Lactones

As allosteric modulators of ionotropic c-aminobutyric acid-(GABA) and glutamate gated chloride channels (GluCl), Macrocyclic Lactones, such as Ivermectin (IVM) and Moxidectin (MOX), rapidly gained popularity in the control of parasitosis. MLs are broad spectrum drugs which display good efficiency against nematodes and arthropods with relatively low toxicity to mammals (Lynagh and Lynch, 2012).

IVM binds irreversibly to GABA receptors of both vertebrates and invertebrates (Campbell, 1985) and GluCl channels of invertebrates (Cully et al., 1994; Arena et al., 1992, Janssen et al., 2013). These channels are assembled by individual *cys*-loop receptor subunits that comprise an extracellular N-terminal ligand-binding domain and four membrane-spanning helices. They can assemble as homomeric or heteromeric pentamers.

In nematodes, GluCl channels are more important targets than the GABA-gated chloride channels. These channels can be activated by ivermectin at concentrations as low as 100 pM and 1uM, respectively (Shan et al., 2001, McCavera et al., 2009) Binding of IVM to the channel causes an irreversible opening which is followed by influx of chloride ions resulting in the hyperpolarization of the neuronal or muscular membranes (Dent et al., 1997). As a result, the drug causes an inhibition of the transmembrane currents, especially on the pharyngeal muscle cells and motor neurons, causing death by paralysis or starvation (Gill et al., 1995, Wolstenholme and Rogers, 2005, Ardelli et al., 2009). A more detailed description of ivermectin action mechanism has been reviewed elsewhere (Yates et al., 2003).

The success of ML led to a wide use throughout the world and inevitably to resistance. There is evidence that selection for IVM resistance can occur within few generations (James and Davey, 2009; Coles et al., 2005; Van Wyk and Malan, 1988). The candidate gene strategy has also been applied to investigate the genetics to ML resistance but, differently from benzimidazoles, has demonstrated a much more complex scenario where multiple loci can be involved in different mechanisms (Table 2). In *H. contortus*, to date, there are at least six GluCl channels genes that code for at least seven subunits. These subunits can assemble into pharmacologically slightly diverse channels that may vary in IVM susceptibility (reviewed by Glendinning et al., 2011). The evidence is that IVM gates the GluCl channel by binding to the alpha-subunit and not the beta-subunit (Cully et al., 1994).

As a classical model used for nematode biology and genetics, *C. elegans* has been used to study the genetic aspects of drug resistance as individual heterologous transporter subunits can be relatively easily cloned and expressed. Chronic exposure to gradually increasing IVM concentrations can select for genetically stable *C. elegans* strains with significantly increased resistance to IVM (James and Davey, 2009).

In *C. elegans*, simultaneous mutations at *avr-14*, *avr-15*, and *glc-1* confers high level resistance to IVM (Dent 2000). As was shown by Glendinning (2011), the GluCl subunit *Hco-glc-2* does not form an IVM sensitive channel while *Hco-acr-14* is capable of forming an IVM sensitive channel when expressed in transgenic *C. elegans*. In addition, in *H. contortus*, it was demonstrated changes in allele frequencies of GluCl subunits because of ivermectin selection (Blackhall et al. 1998).

The importance of GluCl channels was also demonstrated for *C. oncophora* genes expressed in *Xenopus laevis* oocytes. GluCla cDNAs, differing by three non-synonymous substitutions, were cloned from IVM resistant and IVM sensitive *C. oncophora* strains and expressed in *X. laevis* oocytes (Njue et al., 2004). The GluCl-alpha from the resistant strain was 2.5-fold less sensitive to IVM on whole cell voltage clamp recordings. Site-directed mutagenesis experiments suggested that just one of the three substitutions (L256F) was responsible for the loss of sensitivity. Also, this particular polymorphism has yet to be validated for other species of nematodes (Gilleard, 2006).

Although experimental data show that mutation on GluCl genes may provide some level of tolerance to MLs, binding assays fail to relate any consistent changes in IVM binding to *H. contortus* and *T. circumcincta* (Paiement et al., 1999; Hejmadi et al., 2000). This suggests a different mechanism of resistance to ML where mutations of the drug targets may not be as essential as for BZs. In fact there are experimental evidences that suggests a more important role for a gene family that encode for ATP-binding cassettes (ABC transporters), specially p-glycoproteins transporter (*Pgp*).

Pgps are commonly associated with drug transport. The protein pumps the drug out of the cell and therefore prevents from it ever reaching its target. For that reason, these genes, frequently work as multidrug resistance genes. In the first reports that associated ML-resistance in nematodes with ABC transporters, higher pgp expression levels or changes in allelic diversity were documented in resistant *H. contortus* worms (Blackhall et al., 1998; Xu et al., 1998). So far, at least 9 *pgp* genes were described in *H. contortus* (Lespine et al., 2008; Williamson et al., 2011) and 11 partial *pgp* sequences were recently identified in *Teladorsagia circumcincta* (Dicker et al., 2011).

Experimental data strongly suggest that ML resistance can be correlated to both changes in *pgp* expression levels and the alleles involved, not only in *Trichostrongylidae* but also in other worm models. In *H. contortus,* a higher expression of expression of *pgps* was correlated with IVM resistance (Blackhall et al., 1998; Xu et al., 1998).

Later, it was shown, *in vivo*, a higher expression of *pgp-11* in an IVM resistant *H. contortus* population (Prichard and Roulet, 2007). The same was observed in *C. oncophora.* A three to five fold increase in *pgp-11* expression, was described in MOX and IVM exposed adult worms (De Graef et al., 2013). Additionally, constitutive up-regulation *pgp-2* and *pgp-9* was observed in a triple-resistant *H. contortus* isolate (Williamson et al., 2011)

The importance of mutations in the coding regions of *pgps* for the development of ML resistance in trichostrongylids is still unclear. However, it was observed an increase in IVM susceptibility in individual strains of *C. elegans* that carries mutated *pgps* (*pgp-14*, *pgp-11*, *pgp-8*, *pgp-1*, *pgp-12*, *pgp-9* and *pgp-3*). In *C. elegans*, *Pgp-11* and *Pgp-14* were found to be the most important for IVM detoxification (Janssen et al., 2013).

Another interesting aspect of ML resistance is an apparently indirect selection pressure imposed upon the beta-tubulin gene. This was initially reported in *H. contortus* strains treated with IVM or MOX. Similarly, in parasites treated with BZ, a difference in allele frequency was observed in the beta-subunit of the GluCl (Blackhall et al., 1999, Eng et al., 2006). Later this was shown in strains and field isolates of *H. contortus* resistant to IVM and/or MOX (Mottier and Prichard, 2008).

However, the correlation of the resistance mechanisms for both drug families and/or any link between beta-tubulin and any other locus in the ML pathways are not yet very clear (Prichard, 2007).

Tetrahydropyrimidines and Imidazothiazoles

Together with BZ and ML, another class of drugs takes place as key alternative to control of nematode infections, the cholinergic agonists Imidazothiazoles and Tetrahydropyrimidines. Among these, the most important are pyrantel, levamisole, bephenium and monepantel (Aceves et al., 1970; Aubry et al., 1970; Martin et al., 2005).

Most of the known mechanisms of resistance to this class of drugs are related to changes in gene expression such as up/down regulation of targets and expression of alternative spliced isoforms of the drug target (Table 2).

Cholinergic drugs mimic the acetylcholine neurotransmitter and activates the acetylcholine receptors (AChR) of the worm somatic muscles (Martin et al., 2005). Because it is not broken down fast enough, the drug causes a high and long lasting activation of the muscles that result in a spastic paralysis of the nematode, resulting in death and expulsion from the host (Robertson and Martin, 1993). These receptors are classified by its response to LEV (l-AChR), nicotine (nAChR) or bephenium (bAChR) (Martin and Robertson, 2007).

The first registered appearance of levamisole and pyrantel resistance was in 1979 and 1996, respectively (Sangster et al., 1979; Chapman et al., 1996; Kaplan, 2004). Like for ML, much of the current knowledge of mode of action and resistance mechanisms was built based on the model organism *C. elegans*. In this model, resistance to LEV was first associated with three genes, *unc-29*, *unc-38* and *lev-1* (Fleming et al., 1997). Like GluCl receptors, AChR are assembled with two or more alpha subunits and three non-alpha subunits (beta, gamma or delta subunits).

For developmental and physiological reasons, different subunits and its combinations are restricted to particular nerve cells or muscles cells. Also the sensitivity of the channel to the drug may vary depending on its composition, therefore, varying between tissues.

The bephenium sensitive AChR subtype b-AChR is still not well known and most of the studies concerning the role of these receptors on drug resistance are focused on L-AChR subtypes. In *H. contortus*, *T. circumcincta* and *T. colubriformis*, the orthologues of *C. elegans unc-29*, *unc-63*, *unc-38*, *lev-1* and *acr-8* were identified to form the L-AChRs (Hoekstra et al., 1997; Neveu et al., 2010; Walker et al., 2001; Wiley et al., 1996, Fauvin et al., 2010). In *H. contortus*, the assembly of *unc-29.1*, *unc-38*, *unc-63*, *acr-8* forms a LEV sensitive receptor that is less sensitive to acetylcholine (L-AchR1). The exclusion of *acr-8* leads to the formation of a bephenium insensitive receptor that is less sensitive to LEV then to pyrantel (L-AChR2) (Charvet et al., 2012). Also, expression on *acr-8b*, a truncated isoform of *acr-8* can be detected in the resistant UGA/2004 *H. contortus* strain (Williamson et al., 2011).

In *H. contortus, T. circumcincta*, and *T. colubriformis*, expression of *unc-38*, *unc-63*, *unc-29*, and *lev-1* homologs seems to not vary in resistant isolates. However, expression of an abbreviated isoform of *unc-63* (*unc-63b*), that confers some level of resistance to LEV, is enhanced (Neveu et al., 2010; Fauvin et al., 2010).

Together with changes in gene expression, resistance to imidazothiazoles and tetrahydropyrimidines may result from mutations on its targets, although very little is known about the gene mutations associated with the resistant phenotype. In *C. elegans,* null mutations on the *unc-38*, *unc-29* and *unc-63* confers resistance to LEV, while null mutation on the *acr-16* gene confers resistance to nicotine with no effect on LEV resistance (Fleming et al., 1997). The main issue here is the relevance of these mutations on a parasitic nematode, since the impact on the worm fitness is different in a free living nematode such as *C. elegans* and parasitic nematodes that needs to overcome a harsh environment to infect the mammal host and complete its cycle.

Amino-Acetonitrile Derivatives

Recently, a new promising class of drugs was introduced, the Amino-Acetonitrile derivatives (AADs). This is a particularly interesting drug family because the report of resistance and resistance mechanism came short after its release (Table 2).

The Monepantel (MPTL) is an AAD drug that allosterically activates the DEG-3 and DES-2 channels (nAChR) (Rufener et al., 2010). Monepantel have low toxicity to mammals and is active against drug resistant isolates of *H. contortus*, *T. circumcincta* and *T. colubriformis* causing death by paralysis (Kaminsky et al., 2008a; b).

Although it also targets AChR channels, MPTL activates a different subset of channels than LEV, being the preferable targets the DEG-3 and DES-2 subunits present in nAChR channels, while LEV activates l-AChR channels.

Although AADs were recently introduced, resistance has been already documented and characterized. Resistance to MPTL, at least in *H. contortus,* seems to be due to mis-splicing and point mutations in nAChR genes from the DEG-3 subfamily, with particular importance to the mptl1 (acr-23H) locus (Rufener et al., 2009).

Although resistance to ADDs was rapidly identified, this new class of drug takes place as an indispensable alternative to the control of parasitic nematodes.

This is shown in alternative strategies where a mixture of different drug classes is used to minimize the impact of drug resistance in scenario where it is a growing problem (Dobson et al., 2011).

Table 2. Molecular mechanisms associated with ATH drug resistance in trichostronghylid nematodes

Drug Class	Common drugs	Mechanism of action	Resistance mechanism	Genes involved/ Markers of resistance
Benzimidazoles	Mebendazole Oxibendazole Albendazole	Binding to beta-tubulin causes an inhibition of the polymerization of microtubules.	Mutation of target gene.	*Beta-tubulin 1* SNPs: *F200Y, F167Y and E198A.*
Macrocyclic Lactones	Avermectins (Ivermectin)	The drug binds irreversibly to ionotropic c-aminobutyric acid (GABA) and/or glutamate-gated chloride channels (GluCl) receptors causing the opening of the flacid paralysis of pharyngeal and motor muscles of the nematode.	Resistance to ivermectins is usually associated with mutations or changes in expression profiles of the genes that encode subunits of the drug target receptors and also due to mutations and/or up-regulation of ATP-binding cassete genes. Also, beta-tubulin was related to resistance.	*Cooperia spp.*: *GluCla* (L256F), *pgp-11* (up-regulation). *Haemonchus* spp.: *pgp-2* (up-regulation), *pgp-9* (up-regulation).
Imidazothiazoles and Tetrahydropyrimidines	Pyrantel Levamisole Bephenium Moxidectin	The drug binds to nicotinic acetylcholine receptors of the nematode's somatic muscles acting as agonists. The drugs cause rigid paralysis of the nematode.	Changes in the expression patterns of the channels subunits such as changes in expression levels and expression of splicing variants.	*acr-8, unc-63, Hco-mptl-1, Hco-des-2H, unc-29, unc-38, lev-1.*
Amino-Acetonitrile Derivatives	Monepantel	Acivation of AChR channels. The drug causes paralysis if the worm in a manner similar to Cholinergic anthelmintcs.	Mutation or mis-splicing of target genes.	DEG-3 and DES-2 gene family such *as mptl-1* gene.

Dynamics of Anti-Helminthic Resistance Rise and Spread in *Trichoestrongylidae*

From the genetic point of view, the phenomenon of ATH resistance rise can be described as the selective elimination of ATH susceptibility conferring alleles from the nematode population by multiple rounds of drug treatment. This process gradually increases, generation after generation, the relative frequency of pre-existent ATH resistance conferring alleles in the parasite population. Therefore, characteristics from the parasite, the host and the environment, such as those described earlier in this chapter (Table 1) influence the dynamics of ATH resistance rise and spread and must be taken in consideration for the design of rational and sustainable management schemes.

Several reports describe high levels of polymorphisms within trichostrongylid worm populations (Dame et al., 1993, Blouin et al., 1995, Braisher et al., 2004, Silvestre et al., 2009; Archie & Ezenwa, 2011, Brasil et al., 2012). This great genetic variation is thought to be a consequence of high mutation rates coupled with a large effective population size, which may become huge as a consequence of the frequent gene flow among parasite subpopulations from different herds/farms (Blouin et al., 1995). For example, it is estimated that *H. contortus* mitochondrial DNA mutation rate is ten times higher than that usually found among vertebrates (Prichard, 2001). Furthermore, the effective trichostrongylid population sizes are usually enormous because of their high prolificacy, large susceptible host population sizes and high migration rates. Therefore, it is not surprisingly that reports describing ATH resistance in *H. contortus* species are abundant. *H. contortus* females are highly prolific and can produce up to 10.000 eggs per day (Table 1). This parasitic species also possess a broad range of susceptible domestic hosts bred in large herds/flocks worldwide (Table 1). In addition, the frequent host movement, especially among commercial farms, promotes high gene flow among *H. contortus* subpopulations, thereby, enhancing the chances of spread of ATH resistance conferring alleles (Blouin et al., 1995, Prichard, 2001, Brasil et al., 2012). All these factors contribute to increase the likelihood of pre-existence of resistance conferring alleles in the population and the appearance/acquisition of novel/recurrent mutations (Otsen et al., 2000; Brasil et al., 2012). Indeed, there are several reports describing that resistance can originate through different ways such as animal movement among farms (Blouin et al., 1995, Braisher et al., 2004, Cerutti et al., 2010) and novel/recurrent mutations (Silvestre et al., 2009; Skuce et al., 2010; Brasil et al., 2012) in trichostrongylids.

While characteristics from the parasitic species and host movement aforementioned mainly influence the chances of ATH resistance appearance and spread, the rate of ATH resistance rise is particularly influenced by the host susceptibility/chemoprophylaxis regimen and environmental factors. This occurs because the later factors greatly influence the fraction of the nematode populations that are in *refugia* (e.g., eggs and larvae in the pasture, inside asymptomatic/untreated animals or inside animals of other host species), thus not submitted to drug selection. Therefore, populations in *refugia* can function as "buffers" to the drug's selective pressure and slow the process of resistance rise (Prichard, 2001). In line with this, environmental parameters, such as humidity and temperature, influence the proportion of the total population exposed to treatment by altering the number of individuals that are in the pasture in the form of eggs and larvae (Waller, 1997).

Host species susceptibility and chemoprophylaxis regimen also play an important role in the rate of resistance rise. These can be inferred, for example, by the fewer reported cases of resistance in trichostrongylids of cattle compared to small ruminants, such as sheep and goats (Prichard, 2001; Coles et al., 2002). In many cattle enterprises, adult animals remain untreated since they are often resistant (or tolerant) to nematode infections. This alleviates the selective pressure for resistance imposed upon the nematode population by keeping subpopulations under *refugia* inside asymptomatic/untreated animals (Coles et al., 2002). In line with this hypothesis, the prevalence of resistance is highest in ruminants such as goats, where the selection process occurs more intensively due to their relatively poor ability to regulate gastrointestinal nematodes. Indeed, it is a common practice to treat all age classes of non-dairy breeds on a frequent basis. Bioavailability may also be limited in goats by the high incidence of rumen by-pass (Sangster et al., 1991) and the relatively short half-life enjoyed by drugs in the broad-spectrum families (Galtier et al. 1981; Bogan et al., 1987). Additionally, the pathogenicity capacity of each parasite species infection is different and the host–parasite relationships should be considered. Infection with pathogenic worms often requires treatment to control disease, so selection pressure could be higher for these parasites. Indeed, ATH resistance reports are more common for *H. contortus* species infecting small ruminants than for *Cooperia* spp. or even *H. placei* infecting cattle (Prichard, 2001; Coles et al., 2002; Brasil et al., 2012).

Therefore, the multiple factors described in here should be considered when planning strategies for the rational control of trichostrongylids.

For example, quarantine regimens to prevent the host-mediated spread of resistance-associated alleles among farms should be used. This practice should be coupled with treatment with a different drug that has not been routinely used in the incoming herd/animal. The use of directed treatment methods, like FAMACHA®, can also reduce the selective pressure imposed upon the entire nematode population and slow resistance rise. In addition, it is generally preferable to use short-acting drugs to prevent worms being exposed to the sub-therapeutic concentrations that result from an extended half-life of a drug. In experimental studies it was shown that repeated sub-therapeutic treatments with MLs can lead to resistant nematode populations of sheep (Ranjan et al., 2002) and cattle (Molento et al., 1999; Van Zeveren et al., 2007). In the future, the application of molecular tests to screen farm incoming animals for the identity of their parasitic burdens and for the alleles that confer resistance to drugs will aid the development of rational control strategies. Since most of the genetic variability in trichostrongylids is found within hosts, screening of one or a few representative animals from a herd can be informative and should certainly be economically viable. Therefore, combined efforts should be focused on the elucidation of the basis of ATH resistance in order to enable the development of sensitive, specific and cost-effective molecular diagnostic tests.

Conclusion

Antiparasitic drugs undertake a pivotal role in animal welfare and correspond to a significant element in animal production with impact not only in animal health but also in production costs. For this reason, anti-helminthics have been broadly used, frequently decoupled from any other parasite control strategy, which led drug resistance to become a growing problem that threatens animal production throughout the world.

The majority of the anthelmintic resistance cases reported in livestock involves infections with worms from the *Trichostrongylidae* family, mostly from the genera *Haemonchus*, *Trichostrongylus*, *Cooperia* and *Teladorsagia*. To overcome this problem, new strategies of parasite control must take place and for that, a deep understanding of the molecular mechanisms are required to allow the development of early and sensitive detection of resistance, even before it becomes a problem, so the cost of use of anthelmintics can be reduced along with an increase of treatment efficacy. In the future, molecular tests will allow the early detection of resistance and aid the rational and sustainable control of drug resistance.

Acknowledgments

Rafael Assis, Eduardo Bastianetto and Denise Oliveira are CNPq fellowship recipients. Livia Santos is a CAPES fellowship recipient. This work was supported by CNPq (process number INCT 573899/2008-8 and 482852/2011-9) and FAPEMIG (process number INCT APQ-0084/08).

References

Aceves, J.; Erliji, D.; Martinez-Marnon, R. (1970). The mechanism of the paralysing action of tetramisole on Ascaris somatic muscle. *Brit. J. Pharm., 38*, 602-607.

Anziani, O. S., Suarez, V., Guglielmone, A. A., Warnke, O., Grande, H., Coles, G. C., (2004). Resistance to benzimidazole and macrocyclic lactone anthelmintics in cattle nematodes in Argentina. *Vet. Parasitol., 122*, 303–306.

Archie E. A. & Ezenwa, V. O. (2011). Population genetic structure and history of a generalist parasite infecting multiple sympatric host species. *Int. J. Parasitol., 41*, 89–98.

Ardelli, B. F.; Stitt, L. E.; Tompkins, J. B.; Prichard, R. K. (2009). A comparison of the effects of ivermectin and moxidectin on the nematode *Caenorhabditis elegans*. *Vet. Parasitol., 165*, 96–108.

Arena, J. P.; Liu, K. K.; Paress, P.S; Cully, D. F. (1992). Expression of a glutamate-activated chloride current in Xenopus oocytes injected with *Caenorhabditis elegans* RNA: evidence for modulation by avermectin. *Mol. Brain Res., 15,* 339–348.

Artho, R.; Schnyder, M.; Kohler, L.; Torgerson, P. R.; Hertzberg, H. (2007). Avermectin-resistance in gastrointestinal nematodes of Boer goats and Dorper sheep in Switzerland. *Vet. Parasitol. 144*, 68–73.

Aubry, M. L.; Cowell, P.; Davey, M. J.; Shevde, S. (1970). Aspects of the pharmacology of new anthelmintics: pyrantel. *Brit. J. Pharm., 38*, 332-344.

Besier, R. B., Love, S. C. J. (2003). Anthelmintic resistance in sheep nematodes in Australia: the need for new approaches. *Aust. J. Exp. Agric.* 43, 1383–1391.

Blackhall W. (1999) Genetic variation and multiple mechanisms of anthelmintic resistance in Haemonchus Contortus. PhD Thesis, Institute of Parasitology, McGill University, Canada.

Blackhall, W. J.; Liu, H. Y.; Xu, M.; Prichard, R. K.; Beech, R. N. (1998). Selection at a P-glycoprotein gene in ivermectin- and moxidectin-selected strains of *Haemonchus contortus. Mol. Biochem. Parasitol. 95*, 193–201.

Blackhall, W. J; Liu, H. Y.; Xu, M.; Prichard, R. K.; Beech, R. N. (1998). Selection at a P-glycoprotein gene in ivermectin- and moxidectin-selected strains of *Haemonchus contortus. Mol. Biochem. Parasitol., 95,* 193–201.

Blouin, M. S.; Yowell C. A.; Courtney, C. H.; Dame, J. B. (1995). Host movement and the genetic structure of populations of parasitic nematodes. *Genetics, 141,* 1007-1014.

Blouin, M. S.; Yowell, C. A.; Courtney, C. H.; Dame, J.B. (1995). Host movement and the genetic structure of populations of parasitic nematodes. *Genetics, 141,* 1007–1014.

Bogan, J.; Benoit, E.; Delatour, P. (1987). Pharmacokinetics of oxfendazole in goats: acomparison with sheep. *J. Vet. Pharm. Ther., 10,* 305-309.

Borges, F. A., Rodrigues, D. C., Buzzolini, C., Silva, H. C., Oliveira, G. P., & Costa, A. J. (2005). *Haemonchus placei, Cooperia punctata, C. spatulata,* and *C. pectinata* resistant to ivermectin in bovines. In Proceedings of the 20th International Conference of the World Association for the Advancement of Veterinary Parasitology 20, 74.

Borges, F.A.; Silva, H.C.; Buzzulini, C.; Soares, V.E.; Santos, E.; Oliveira, G.P.; Costa, A.J. (2008). Endectocide activity of a new long-action formulation containing 2.25% ivermectin+1.25% abamectin in cattle. *Vet. Parasitol,. 155*, 299–307.

Braisher, T. L.; Gemmell, N. J.; Grenfell, B. T.; Amos, W. (2004). Host isolation and patterns of genetic variability in three populations of *Teladorsagia* from sheep. *Int. J. Parasitol., 34*, 1197–1204.

Braisher, T.L.; Gemmell, N.J.; Grenfell, B.T.; Amos, W. Host isolation and patterns of genetic variability in three populations of *Teladorsagia* from sheep. (2004). *Int. J. Parasitol., 34,* 1197–1204.

Brasil, B. S. A. F.; Nunes, R. L.; Bastianetto, E.; Drummond, M. G.; Carvalho, D. C.; Leite, R. C.; Molento, M.B.; Oliveira, D. A. A. (2012). Genetic diversity patterns of *Haemonchus placei* and *Haemonchus contortus* populations isolated from domestic ruminants in Brazil. *Internat. J. Parasitol., 42*, 469–479.

Campbell, W. C. (1985). Ivermectin: an update. *Parasitol. Today, 1*, 10-16.

Cerutti, M. C.; Citterio, C. V.; Bazzocchi, C.; Epis, S.; D'Amelio, S.; Ferrari, N.; Lanfranchi, P. (2010). Genetic variability of *Haemonchus contortus* (*Nematoda: Trichostrongyloidea*) in alpine ruminant host species. *J. Helminthol., 84,* 276–283.

Chapman, M.R.; French, D.D.; Monahan, C.M.; Klei, T.R. (1996). Identification and characterization of a pyrantel pamoate resistant cyathostome population. *Vet. Parasitol,. 66,* 205–212.

Charvet, C. L.; Robertson, A. P.; Cabaret, J.; Martin, R. J.; Neveu, C. (2012). Selective effect of the anthelmintic bephenium on *Haemonchus contortus* levamisole-sensitive acetylcholine receptors. *Invert. Neurosci., 12*, 43-51.

Coles, G. C. (2002). Catlle nematodes resistant to anthelmintics: Why so few cases? *Vet. Res., 33,* 481-489.

Coles, G.C. (1986). Anthelmintic resistance in sheep. *Vet. Clin. North Am. Food Anim. Pract., 2*, 423–432.

Coles, G.C. (2005). Anthelmintic resistance –looking to the future: a UK perspective. *Res. Vet. Sci., 78*, 99-108.

Condi, G. K.; Soutello, R. G. V.; Amarante, A. F. T. (2009). Moxidectin-resistant nematodes in cattle in Brazil. *Vet. Parasitol. 161*, 213–217.

Cully, D. F.; Vassilatis, D. K.; Liu, K. K.; Paress, P.; Van der Ploeg, L. H. T.; Schaeffer, J. M.; Arena, J. P. (1994). Cloning of an avermectin-sensitive glutamate-gated chloride channel from *Caenorhabditis elegans*. *Nature, 371*, 707–711.

da Cruz, D. G.; da Rocha, L. O.; Arruda, S. S.; Palieraqui, J. G. B.; Cordeiro, R. C.; Santos Junior, E.; Molento, M. B.; de Paula Santos, O. C. (2010). Anthelmintic efficacy and management practices in sheep farms from the state of Rio de Janeiro, Brazil. *Vet. Parasitol., 170*, 340–343.

Dame, J. B.; Blouin, M. S.; Courtney, C. H. (1993). Genetic structure of populations of *Ostertagia ostertagi*. *Vet. Parasitol., 46,* 55–62.

Davidse, L. C., & Flach, W. (1977). Differential binding of methyl benzimidazol-2-yl carbamate to fungal tubulin as a mechanism of resistance to this antimitotic agent in mutant strains of *Aspergillus nidulans. J. Cell Biol., 72,* 174-193.

De Graef, J.; Demeler, J.; Skuce, P.; Mitreva, M.; Von Samson-Himmelstjerna, G.; Vercruysse, J.; Claerebout, E.; Geldhof, P. (2013). Gene expression analysis of ABC transporters in a resistant *Cooperia oncophora* isolate following in vivo and in vitro exposure to macrocyclic lactones. *Parasitology,140*, 499–508.

Demeler, J.; van Zeveren, A. M. J.; Kleinschmidt, N.; Vercruysse, J.; Ho¨glund, J.; Koopmann, R.; Cabaret, J.; Claerebout, D. P.; Areskog, M.; Von Samson-Himmelstjerna, G. (2009). Monitoring the efficacy of ivermectin and albendazole against gastro intestinal nematodes of cattle in Northern Europe. *Vet. Parasitol., 109,* 109–115.

Dent, J. A.; Davis, M. W.; Avery, L. (1997). avr-15 encodes a chloride channel subunit that mediates inhibitory glutamatergic neurotransmission and ivermectin sensitivity in *Caenorhabditis elegans. EMBO J., 16*, 5867-5879.

Dent, J. A; Smith, M. M; Vassilatis, D. K; Avery, L. (2000). The genetics of avermectin resistance in *Caenorhabditis elegans. Proc. Natl Acad. Sci. U. S. A., 97*, 2674–2679.

Dicker, A. J.; Nisbet, A. J.; Skuce, P. J. (2011). Gene expression changes in a P-glycoprotein (Tci-pgp-9) putatively associated with ivermectin resistance in *Teladorsagia circumcincta. Int. J. Parasitol., 41,* 935–942.

Dobson, R. J.; Hosking, B. C.; Besier, R. B.; Love, S.; Larsen, J. W. A.; Rolfe, P. F.; Bailey, J. N. (2011). Minimising the development of anthelmintic resistance, and optimising the use of the novel anthelmintic monepantel, for the sustainable control of nematode parasites in Australian sheep grazing systems. *Aus. Vet. J., 89*, 160–166.

Edmonds, M. D.; Johnson, E. G.; Edmonds, J. D. (2010). Anthelmintic resistance of *Ostertagia ostertagi* and *Cooperia oncophora* to macrocyclic lactones in cattle from the western United States. *Vet. Parasitol. 170,* 224–229.

Eng, J. K. L.; Blackhall, W. J.; Osei-Atweneboana, M. Y.; Bourguinat, C.; Galazzo, D.; Beech, R. N.; Unnasch, T. R.; Awadzi, K.; Lubega, G. W.; Prichard, R. K. (2006). Ivermectin selection on β-tubulin: Evidence in *Onchocerca volvulus* and *Haemonchus contortus. Mol. Biochem. Parasitol., 150*, 229–235.

Fauvin, A.; Charvet, C.; Issouf, M.; Cortet, J.; Cabaret, J.; Neveu, C. (2010). cDNA-AFLP analysis in levamisole-resistant *Haemonchus contortus* reveals alternative splicing in a nicotinic acetylcholine receptor subunit. *Mol. Biochem. Parasitol., 170*, 105–107.

Fiel, C.A.; Saumell, C.A.; Steffan, P.E.; Rodriguez, E.M. (2001). Resistance of Cooperia to ivermectin treatments in grazing cattle of the Humid Pampa. Argentina. *Vet. Parasitol,. 97*, 211–217.

Fleming, J. T.; Squire, M. D.; Barnes, T. M.; Tornoe, C.; Matsuda, K.; Ahnn, J. Fire, A.; Sulston, J. E.; Barnard, E. A.; Sattelle, D. B.; Lewis, J. A. (1997). *Caenorhabditis elegans* levamisole resistance genes Lev-1, unc-29, and unc-38 encode functional nicotinic acetylcholine receptor subunits. *J. Neuroscience, 17*, 5843-5857.

Galtier, P.; Escoula, L.; Camguilhem, R.; Alvinierie, M. (1981). Comparative bioavailability of levamizole in non lactating ewes and goats. *Ann. Rec. Vet., 12*, 109-115.

Gasbarre, L.C.; Smith, L. L.; Hoberg, E.; Pilitt, P. A. (2009). Further characterisation of a cattle nematode population with demonstrated resistance to current anthelmintics. *Vet. Parasitol., 166,* 275–280

Geary, T. G.; Nulf, S. C.; Favreau, M. A.; Tang, L.; Prichard, R. K.; Hatzenbuhler, N. T.; Shea, M. H.; Alexander, S. J.; Klein, R. D. (1992). Three β-tubulin cDNAs from the parasitic nematode *Haemonchus contortus. Mol. Biochem. Parasitol., 50*, 295–306.

Geary, T. G.; Nulf, S. C.; Favreau, M. A.; Tang, L.; Prichard, R. K.; Hatzenbuhler, N. T.; Shea, M. H.; Alexander, S. J.; Klein, R. D. (1992). Three b-tubulin cDNAs from the parasitic nematode *Haemonchus contortus. Mol. Biochem. Parasitol,. 50*, 295–306.

Ghisi, M.; Kaminsky, R.; Maser, P. (2007). Phenotyping and genotyping of *Haemonchus contortus* isolates reveals a new putative candidate mutation for benzimidazole resistance in nematodes. *Vet. Parasitol. 144,* 313–320.

Gill, J. H.; Redwin, J. M.; van Wyk, J. A.; Lacey, E. (1995). Avermectin inhibition of larval development in *H. contortus* effects of ivermectin resistance. *Int. J. Parasitol., 25*, 463–470.

Gilleard, J.S. (2006). Understanding anthelmintic resistance: the need for genomics and genetics. *Int. J. Parasitol., 36*, 1227–1239.

Glendinning, S. K.; Buckingham, S. D.; Sattelle, D. B.; Wonnacott, S., Wolstenholme, A. J. (2011). Glutamate-Gated Chloride Channels of Haemonchus contortus Restore Drug Sensitivity to Ivermectin Resistant *Caenorhabditis elegans*. PLoS ONE 6(7): e22390. doi:10.1371/journal.pone.0022390

Hejmadi, M. V.; Jagannathan, S.; Delany, N. S.; Coles, G. C; Wolstenholme, A. J. (2000). L-glutamate binding sites of parasitic nematodes: an association with ivermectin resistance? *Parasitology, 120,* 535–545.

Hoekstra, J. W. R; Roos, M. H.; Wiley, L. J.; Weiss, A. S; Sangster, N. C.; Tait, A. (2001). Cloning and structural analysis of partial acetylcholine receptor subunit genes from the parasitic nematode *Teladorsagia circumcincta. Vet. Parasitol., 97*, 329–335.

Hoekstra, R.; Visser, A.; Wiley, L.J.; Weiss, A.S.; Sangster, N.C.; Roos, M.H. (1997) Characterisation of an acetylcholine receptor gene of *Haemonchus contortus* in relation to levamisole resistance. *Mol. Biochem. Parasitol., 84,* 179–187.

Hosking, B.C.; Watson T. G.; Leathwick DM. (1996). Multigeneric resistance to oxfendazole by nematodes in cattle. *Vet. Rec., 138*, 67–68.

Howell, S. B.; Burke, J. M.; Miller, J. E.; Terrill, T. H.; Valencia, E.; Williams, M. J.; Williamson, L. H.; Zajac, A. M.; Kaplan, R. M. (2008). Prevalence of anthelmintic resistance on sheep and goatfarms in the southeastern United States. *J. Am. Vet. Med. Assoc. 233,* 1913–1919.

Jabbar, A.; Iqbal, Z.; Kerboeuf, D.; Muhammad, G.; Khan, M. N.; Afaq, M. (2006). Anthelmintic resistance: The state of play revisited. *Life Sci.,79*, 2413-2431.

Jackson, F. & Coop, R. L. (2000). The development of anthelmintic resistance in sheep nematodes. *Parasitology, 120*, S95-S107.

Jackson, R. A.; Townsenda, K. G.; Pykeb, C.; Lance, D. M. (1987). Isolation of oxfendazole resistant Cooperia oncophora in cattle. *N. Z. Vet. J., 35*, 187–189.

James, C. E. & Davey, M. W. (2009). Increased expression of ABC transport proteins is associated with ivermectin resistance in the model nematode *Caenorhabditis elegans*. *Int. J. Parasitol., 39*, 213–220.

Janssen, I. J. I.; Krücken, J.; Demeler, J.; von Samson-Himmelstjerna, G. (2013). *Caenorhabditis elegans*: Modest increase of susceptibility to ivermectin in individual P-glycoprotein loss-of-function strains. *Exp. Parasitol., 134*, 171–177.

Jeannin, P. C.; Bairden, K.; Gettinby, G.; Murray, M.; Urquhart, G. M. (1990). Efficacy of nitroxynil against ivermectin, benzimidazole and salicylanilide resistant *H. contortus*. *Vet. Rec., 126*, 624–625.

Kaminsky, R.; Ducray, P.; Jung, M.; Clover, R.; Rufener, L.; Bouvier, J.; Weber, S. S.; Wenger, A.; Wieland-Berghausen S.; Goebel T.; Gauvry, N.; Pautrat, F.; Skripsky, T.; Froelich, O.; Komoin-Oka, C.; Westlund, B.; Sluder, A.; Mäser, P. (2008). A new class of anthelmintics effective against drug-resistant nematodes. *Nature, 452*, 176 –180.

Kaminsky, R.; Gauvry, N.; Schorderet, ?; Weber, S.; Skripsky, T.; Bouvier, J.; Wenger, A.; Schroeder, F.; Desaules, Y.; Hotz, R.; Goebel, T., et al. (2008). Identification of the amino-acetonitrile derivative monepantel (AAD 1566) as a new anthelmintic drug development candidate. *Parasitol. Res., 103*, 931–939.

Kaplan, R. M. & Vidyashankarb, N. (2012). An inconvenient truth: Global worming and anthelmintic resistance. *Vet. Parasitol., 186,* 70–78.

Kaplan, R. M. (2004). Drug resistance in nematodes of veterinary importance: a status report. *Trends Parasitol.,20*, 477–481.

Kwa, M. S. G.; Veenstra, J. G.; Roos, M. H. (1993). Molecular characterisation of β-tubulin genes in benzimidazole-resistant populations of *Haemonchus contortus*. *Mol. Biochem. Parasitol., 60,* 133–144.

Kwa, M. S. G.; Kooyman, F. N. J.; Boersema, J. H.; Roos, M. H. (1993). Effect of selection for benzimidazole resistance in Haemonchus contortus on beta-tubulin isotype 1 and isotype 2 genes. *Biochem. Bioph. Res. Co., 191,* 413–419.

Kwa, M. S. G.; Veenstra, J. G.; van Dujk M, Roos, M. H. (1995). Beta-tubulin genes from the parasitic nematode *Haemonchus contortus* modulate drug resistance in *Caenorhabditis elegans*. *J. Mol. Biol., 246,* 500–510.

Lacey, E. & Prichard, R.K. (1986). Interactions of benzimidazoles (BZ) with tubulin from BZ-sensitive and BZ-resistant isolates of *Haemonhus contortus*. *Mol. Biochem. Parasitol., 19*, 171–181.

Lacey, E. & Watson, T. R. (1985) Activity of benzimidazole carbamates against L1210 mouse leukaemia cells: correlation with in vitro tubulin polymerisation assay. *Biochem. Pharmacol., 34*, 3603–3605.

Lacey, E.; Brady, R. L.; Prichard, R. K.; Watson, T. R. (1987). Comparison of inhibition of polymerisation of mammalian tubulin and helminth ovicidal activity by benzimidazole carbamates. *Vet. Parasitol., 23*, 105–119.

Leathwick, D. M.; Moen, I. C.; Miller, C. M.; Sutherland, I. A. (2000). Ivermectin resistant *Ostertagia circumcincta* from sheep in the lower North Island and their susceptibility to other macrocyclic lactone anthelmintics. *N. Z. Vet. J,. 48*, 151–154.

Lespine, A.; Alvinerie, M.; Vercruysse, J.; Prichard, R. K.; Geldhof, P. (2008). ABC transporter modulation: a strategy to enhance the activity of macrocyclic lactone anthelmintics. *Trends in Parasitology, 24,* 293–298.

Love, S. (2007). Drench resistance and sheep worm control. In: Primefact, 478, 1–5.

Loveridge B.; McArthur M.; McKenna, P. B.; Mariadass, B. (2003). Probable multigeneric resistance to macrocyclic lactone anthelmintics in cattle in New Zealand. *N. Z. Vet. J., 51*, 139–141.

Lubega, G. W. & Prichard, R. K. (1991). Interaction of benzimidazole anthelmintics with *Haemonchus contortus* tubulin: binding affinity and anthelmintic efficacy. *Exp. Parasitol., 73,* 203–213.

Lubega, G. W. & Prichard, R. K. (1991). Specific interaction of benzimidazole anthelmintics with tubulin from developing stages of thiabendazole-susceptible and -resistant *Haemonchus contortus*. *Biochem. Pharmacol., 41,* 93–101.

Lyndal-Murphy, M.; Rogers, D.; Ehrlich, W. K.; James, P. J.; Pepper, P. M. (2009). Reduced efficacy of macrocyclic lactone treatments in controlling gastrointestinal nematode infections of weaner dairy calves in subtropical eastern Australia. *Vet. Parasitol. 168,* 146–150.

Lynagh, T.; Lynch, J. W. (2012). Ivermectin binding sites in human and invertebrate Cys-loop receptors. *Trends Pharmacol. Sci., 33,* 432-441.

Martin, R. J. & Robertson, A. P. (2007). Mode of action of levamisole and pyrantel, anthelmintic resistance, E153 and Q57. *Parasitology, 134,* 1093-1104.

Martin, R. J.; Verma, S.; Levandoski, M.; Clark, C. L.; Qian, H.; Stewart, M.; Robertson, A. P. (2005). Drug resistance and neurotransmitter receptors of nematodes: recent studies on the mode of action of levamisole. *Parasitology, 131*, S71-S84.

Mason, P. C. & McKay, C. H. (2006). Field studies investigating anthelmintic resistance in young cattle on five farms in New Zealand. *N.Z. Vet. J., 54,* 318–322.

McCavera S.; Rogers, A. T.; Yates, D. M.; Woods, D. J.; Wolstenholme, A. J. (2009). An ivermectin-sensitive glutamate-gated chloride channel from the parasitic nematode, *Haemonchus contortus. Mol. Pharmacol., 75,* 1347–1355.

McCracken, R. O. & Stillwell, W. H. (1991). A possible biochemical mode of action for benzimidazole anthelmintics. *Int. J. Parasitol., 21,* 99–104.

McKenna, P. B. (1991). Resistance to benzimidazole anthelmintics in cattle in New Zealand. *N. Z. Vet. J., 39*, 154–155.

Molento, M. B. & Prichard, R. K. (1999). Effects of the multidrug-resistance-reversing agents verapamil and CL 347,099 on the efficacy of ivermectin or moxidectin against unselected and drug-selected strains of *Haemonchus contortus* in jirds (Meriones unguiculatus). *Parasitol. Res., 85*, 1007-1011.

Molento, M. B.; Fortes, F. S.; Pondelek, D.A.S.; Borges, F.A.; Chagas, A. C. S.; Torres-Acosta, J. F.; Geldhof, P. (2011). Challenges of nematode controlin ruminants: focus on Latin America. *Vet. Parasitol,. 180*, 126–132.

Mottier, M. L. & Prichard, R. K. (2008). Genetic analysis of a relationship between macrocyclic lactone and benzimidazole anthelmintic selection on *Haemonchus contortus*. *Pharmacogenet. Genomics, 18*, 129-140.

Neveu, C.; Charvet, C. L.; Fauvin, A.; Cortet, J.; Beech, R. N.; Cabaret, J. (2010). Genetic diversity of levamisole receptor subunits in parasitic nematode species and abbreviated transcripts associated with resistance. *Pharmacogenet. Genomics*, *20*, 414-425.

Njue, A. I. & Prichard, R. K. (2003). Cloning two full-length beta-tubulin isotype cDNAs from *Cooperia oncophora*, and screening for benzimidazole resistance-associated mutations in two isolates. *Parasitology, 127*, 579–588.

Njue, A. I.; Hayashi, J.; Kinne, L.; Feng, X-P., Prichard, R. K. (2004). Mutations in the extracellular domain of glutamate-gated chloride channel α3 and β subunits from ivermectin-resistant *Cooperia oncophora* affect agonist sensitivity. *J. Neurochem.*, *89*, 1137–1147.

Nunes, R. L., dos Santos, L. L., Bastianetto, E., de Oliveira, D. A. A., & Brasil, B. S. A. F. (2013) Frequency of benzimidazole resistance in Haemonchus contortus populations isolated from buffalo, goat and sheep herds. *Revista Brasileira de Parasitologia Veterinária*, *22*, 548-553.

Otsen, M.; Plas, M. E.; Lenstra, J. A.; Roos, M. H.; Hoekstra, R. (2000). Microsatellite diversity of isolates of the parasitic nematode *Haemonchus contortus*. *Mol. Biochem. Parasitol., 110*, 69–77.

Paiement, J. P.; Leger, C.; Ribeiro, P.; Prichard, R. K. (1999). *Haemonchus contortus:* effects of glutamate, ivermectin, and moxidectin on inulin uptake activity in unselected and ivermectin-selected adults. *Exp. Parasitol., 92*, 193–198.

Paiement, J.P.; Prichard, R. K.; Ribeiro, P. (1999). Haemonchus contortus: Characterizationof a glutamate binding site in unselected and ivermectin-selected larvae and adults. *Exp. Parasitol., 92*, 32–39.

Papadopoulos, E. (2008). Anthelmintic resistance in sheep nematodes. *Small Rumin. Res., 76*, 99–103.

Prichard, R. (1990). Anthelmintic resistance in nematodes: extent, recent understanding and future directions for control and research. *Int. J. Parasitol., 20*, 515–523.

Prichard, R. (2001). Genetic variability following selection of *Haemonchus contortus* with anthelmintics. *Trends Parasitol., 17*, 445–453.

Prichard, R. K. & Roulet, A. (2007). ABC transporters and beta-tubulin in macrocyclic lactone resistance: prospects for marker development. *Parasitology, 134,* 1123–1132.

Prichard, R. K.; Hall, C. A.; Kelly, J. D.; Martin, I. C. A.; Donald, A. D. (1980). The problem of anthelmintic resistance in nematodes. *Aust. Vet. J., 56*, 239–251.

Prichard, R.K. (2007). Markers for benzimidazole resistance in human parasitic nematodes? *Parasitology, 134*, 1087–1092.

Ranjan, S.; Wang, G. T; Hirschlein, C.; Simkins, K. L (2002). Selection for resistance to macrocyclic lactones by *Haemonchus contortus* in sheep. *Vet. Parasitol., 103*, 109–117.

Robertson, S.J. & Martin, R.J. (1993). Levamisole-activated single-channel currents from muscle of the nematode parasite *Ascaris suum. Brit. J. Pharm., 108*, 170–178.

Roos, M. H.; Boersema, J. H.; Borgsteede, F. H. M.; Cornelissen, J.; Taylor, M.; Ruitenberg, E. J. (1990). Molecular analysis of selection for benzimidazole resistance in the sheep parasite *Haemonchus contortus. Mol. Biochem. Parasitol., 43*, 77–88

Rufener, L.; Baur, R.; Kaminsky, R.; Ma¨ ser, P.; Sigel, E. (2010). Monepantel Allosterically Activates DEG-3/DES-2 Channels of the Gastrointestinal Nematode *Haemonchus contortus. Mol. Pharmacol., 78,* 895–902.

Rufener, L.; Kaminsky, R.; Maser, P. (2009). In vitro selection of *Haemonchus contortus* for benzimidazole resistance reveals a mutation at amino acid 198 of beta-tubulin. *Mol. Biochem. Parasitol., 168*, 120–122.

Sangster, N. C.; Whitlock, H. V.; Russ, I. G.; Gunawan, M.; Griffin, D.L.; Kelly, J. D. (1979). *Trichostrongylus colubriformis* and *Ostertagia circumcincta* resistant to levamisole, morantel tartrate and thiabendazole: occurrence of field strains. *Res. Vet. Sci., 27,* 106–110.

Sargison, N. D.; Jackson, F.; Wilson, D. J.; Bartley, D. J.; Penny, C. D.; Gilleard, J. S. (2010). Characterisation of milbemycin-, avermectin-, imidazothiazole- and benzimidazole-resistant *Teladorsagia circumcincta* from a sheep flock. *Vet. Rec., 166,* 681–686.

Saunders, G.I.; Wasmuth, J. D.; Beech, R.; Laing, R.; Hunt, M.; Naghra, H.; Cotton, J. A.; Berriman, M.; Britton, C.; Gilleard, J. S. (2013). Characterization and comparative analysis of the complete *Haemonchus contortus* β-tubulin gene family and implications for benzimidazole resistance in strongylid nematodes. *Int. J. Parasitol., 43*, 465–475.

Schnyder, M.; Torgerson, P. R.; Schonmann, M.; Kohler, L.; Hertzberg, H. (2005). Multiple anthelmintic resistance in *Haemonchus contortus* isolated from South African Boer goats in Switzerland. *Vet. Parasitol., 128,* 285–290.

Scott, E. W. & Armour, J. (1991). Effect of development of resistance to benzimidazoles, salicylanilides and ivermectin on the pathogenicity and survival of *Haemonchus contortus. Vet. Rec.,128*, 346-349.

Sczesny-Moraes, E. A.; Bianchin, I.; da Silva, K. F.; Catto, J. B.; Honer, M. R.; Paiva, F. (2010). Anthelmintic resistance of gastrointestinal nematodes in sheep, Mato Grosso do Sul, Brazil. *Pesqui. Vet. Bras.*, *30*, 229–236.

Shan, Q.; Haddrill, J. L.; Lynch, J. W. (2001) Ivermectin, an Unconventional Agonist of the Glycine Receptor Chloride Channel. *J. Biol. Chem., 276*, 12556-12564.

Silvestre, A.; Cabaret, J.; Humbert, J. F. (2001). Effect of benzimidazole under-dosing on the resistant allele frequency in *Teladorsagia circumcincta* (Nematoda). *Parasitology, 123*, 103–111.

Silvestre, A.; Sauve, C.; Cortet, J.; Cabaret, j. (2009). Contrasting genetic structures of two parasitic nematodes, determined on the basis of neutral microsatellite markers and selected anthelmintic resistance markers. *Mol. Ecol., 18,* 5086–5100.

Skuce, P.; Stenhouse, L.; Jackson, F.; Hypša, V.; Gilleard. J. (2010). Benzimidazole resistance allele haplotype diversity in United Kingdom isolates of *Teladorsagia circumcincta* supports a hypothesis of multiple origins of resistance by recurrent mutation. *Int. J. Parasitol., 40,* 1247–1255.

Stafford, K. & Coles, G.C. (1999). Nematode control practices and anthelmintic resistance in dairy calves in the south west of England. *Vet. Rec., 144,* 659–661.

Suarez, V. H. & Cristel, S. L. (2007). Anthelmintic resistance in cattle nematode in the western Pampeana Region of Argentina. *Vet. Parasitol., 144*, 111–117.

Sutherland, I. A. & Leathwick, D. M. (2011). Anthelmintic resistance in nematode parasites of cattle: a global issue? *Trends Parasitol., 27,* 176–181.

van Wyk, J. A. & Malan, F. S. (1988). Resistance of field strains of *Haemonchus contortus* to ivermectin, closantel, rafoxanide and the benzimidazoles in South Africa. *Vet. Rec., 123*, 226-228.

Van Wyk, J. A.; Malan, F. S.; Gerber, H.; Alves, R. (1987). Two field strains of *Haemonchus contortus* resistant to rafoxanide. *Onderstepoort J. Vet. Res., 54*, 143–146.

Van Wyk, J. A.; Stenson, M. O.; Van der Merwe, J. S.; Vorster, R. J.; Viljoen, P. G. (1999). Anthelmintic resistance in South Africa: surveys indicate an extremely serious situation in sheep and goat farming. *Onderstepoort J. Vet. Res., 66*, 273–284.

Van Zeveren, A. M.; Visser, A.; Hoorens, P. R.; Vercruysse, J.; Claerebout, E.; Geldhof, P. (2007). Evaluation of reference genes for quantitative real-time PCR in *Ostertagia ostertagi* by the coefficient of variation and geNorm approach. *Mol. Biochem. Parasitol., 153*, 224–227.

Waghorn, T. S.; Leathwick, D. M.; Rhodes, A. P.; Jackson, R.; Pomroy, W. E.; West, D. M.; Moffat, J. R. (2006). Prevalence of anthelmintic resistance on 62 beef cattle farms in the North Island of New Zealand. *N.Z. Vet. J., 54,* 278–282.

Waller, P. J. (1997). Nematode parasite control of livestock in the tropics/subtropics: the need for novel approaches. *Int. J. Parasitol., 27,* 1193–1201.

Waller, P.J. & Prichard, R.K. Drug resistance in nematodes. In: W.C. Campbell, R.S. Rew. *Chemotherapy of Parasitic Diseases*. Plenum Press, 1986, 339–362.

Waller, P.J. (1987). Anthelmintic resistance and the future for roundworm control. *Vet. Parasitol., 25,* 177-191.

Warwick N. Grant, Lisa J. Mascorda (1996). Beta-tubulin gene polymorphism and benzimidazole resistance in *Trichostrongylus colubriformis. Int. J. Parasitol., 26*, 71–77.

Wiley, L. J.; Weiss, A. S.; Sangster, N. C.; Li, Q. (1996). Cloning and sequence analysis of the candidate nicotinic acetylcholine receptor alpha subunit gene tar-1 from *Trichostrongylus colubriformis. Gene, 182*, 97–100.

Williamson, S. M.; Storey, B.; Howell, S; Harper, K. M.; Kaplan, R. M.; Wolstenholme, A. J. (2011). Candidate anthelmintic resistance-associated gene expression and sequence polymorphisms in a triple-resistant field isolate of *Haemonchus contortus. Mol Biochem Parasitol, 180,* 99–105.

Wolstenholme, A. J. & Rogers, A. T. (2005). Glutamate-gated chloride channels and the mode of action of the avermectin/milbemycin anthelmintics. *Parasitology, 131,* S85–S95.

Xu, M.; Molento, M.; Blackhall, W.; Ribeiro, P.; Beech, R.; Prichard, R. (1998). Ivermectin resistance in nematodes may be caused by alteration of P-glycoprotein homolog. *Mol. Biochem. Parasitol. 91*, 327–335.

Yates, D. M.; Portillo, V.; Wolstenholme, A. J. (2003). The avermectin receptors of *Haemonchus contortus* and *Caenorhabditis elegans. Int. J. Parasitol., 33,* 1183–1193.

In: Anthelmintics
Editor: William Quick
ISBN: 978-1-63117-714-9

Chapter 4

Plants from Cerrado for the Control of Gastrointestinal Nematodes of Ruminants

Franciellen Morais-Costa[1], Viviane de Oliveira Vasconcelos[2], Eduardo Robson Duarte[3] and Walter dos Santos Lima[1]

[1]Programa de Pós-graduação em Parasitologia. Instituto de Ciências Biológicas/Universidade Federal de Minas Gerais. Brasil
[2]Departamento de Fisiopatologia. Universidade Estadual de Montes Claros. Minas Gerais. Brasil
[3]Mestrado em Produção Animal. Instituto de Ciências Agrárias/Universidade Federal de Minas Gerais. Brasil

Abstract

The gastrointestinal helminthes are major limiting factors for the sheep and goat production in the world and the health of livestock depends of effective control of nematodes. The constant administration and inadequate doses of chemical anthelmintics favors the selection of resistant populations and residues these products contribute to the contamination of animal products and of the ambient. The use of herbal treatment in veterinary medicine is a promising field of research. Studies in this area require the insertion into an agroecological context, with the limiting factor to the sustainable management of natural resources involved. The phytotherapy for the parasite control is an alternative that can reduce the cost with the purchase of anthelmintics as well, preventing the emergence of anthelmintic resistance and residues in animal products. Plant species that have tannins in its constitution are known to possess anthelmintic activity, requiring, however, that their efficacies are scientifically proven. The Cerrado is an import biome with high diversity of plants rich in tannins and other metabolic with potential anthelmintic effect. This study presents a review of research on plant species, tested in the Cerrado for the control of helminths in ruminants.

Keywords: Anthelmintic, nematodes, medicinal plants, Cerrado, ruminants

Introduction

The main problem in the small ruminants and limiting of economic exploitation is the gastrointestinal parasites. *Haemonchus contortus* is a nematode of abomasum and feeds of blood throughout, with high prevalence and high pathogenicity (Strong, 1993). Sheep with haemoncoses may show anemia and submandibular edema, with high mortality in young lambs and females in peripartum. Both sexes at all age levels may be intensely affected, reducing weight gain and reproductive capacity, as well as milk, wool, and hide production (Bizimenyera et al., 2006).

The treatment with anthelmintics has been intensely used to control by breeders. The constant administration and the inadequate dosages can favor the selection of the parasite populations resistant to the anthelmintics and contributes to the contamination of animal products with residues of these products (Amarante et al., 1992).

The main anthelmintics were developed during the 60's and are actually essential to control of nematodes. There are currently only three groups of broad spectrum anthelmintics and two groups of small spectrum used to control these parasites (Amarante et al., 1992). Early studies reported resistant helminthes to the group of benzimidazole and levamisoles. With the discovery of a chemical group distinct anthelmintic, avermectins, was represented an alternative treatment with a potent drug for the nematode control in domestic animals (Gopal et al., 1999). Multi-resistant nematodes have been found on several ruminant herds (Molento and Prichard 2001; Taylor et al., 2009; Wolstenholme et al., 2004; Thomaz-Soccol et al., 2004). The possibility of anthelminthic residues in the environment and in animals reared for consumption (Hammond et al., 1997), as well as the spread of multi-resistant strains demands research into alternatives for gastrointestinal nematodes (GIN) control.

The utilization of plants containing secondary compounds such as condensed tannins may expand the organic alternatives to controlling GINs (Athanasiadou et al., 2007; Kahn and Diaz-Hernandez 2000). Phytotherapy in the control of parasitism is an alternative that can reduce the cost with the purchase of anthelmintics, and prevent the emergence of anthelmintic resistance and the presence of residues in animal products. Many plants are traditionally known as having anthelmintic activity, requiring, however, that their efficacy be scientifically proven (Vieira, 2003). Scientific validation of the anthelminthic effects and possible side-effects of plant products is necessary prior to their adoption as novel methods for control (Githiori et al., 2006).

The Cerrado biome, which covers 5% of the world flora, is the second largest source of biodiversity in Brazil (Sano, 2008). However, much of the native vegetation has been destroyed and many species are threatened of extinction, which would enable a wide use and maintenance of food, medicinal, ornamental, linseed and tannin production.

However, few studies have evaluated the anthelmintic effect of the plant species of the Cerrado for the control of GNI. Therefore, the analysis of potential plant species of this biome for helminthes control for ruminants may represent a promising strategy for the biotechnology industry and consequently for the breeders of these animals.

The Cerrado

Among the vegetation types that cover the American continent, the Cerrado presents a natural grandeur of plant species, which demonstrates the importance of education for the conservation and management of this biome. The original vegetation of the Cerrado has already been reduced by over 37 % (Felfili et al., 2002), prejudicing much of its biodiversity. Mittermeier et al. (1999) estimated that 67 % of the Cerrado areas are considered “highly modified” and only 20 % are in original condition, since the changes began with the colonization process, with the introduction of cattle, associated with rudimentary agricultural practices (Zanetti, 1994).

According Eiten (1993), the Cerrado's flora is composed of two groups of species: thick stem trees and bushes with an undergrowth layer, consisting in a large mosaic, which includes a forest canopy formation more or less closed, containing trees with heights of 12 m tall or more. It has a woodland category, usually around six or seven meters and undergrowth stratum more or less continuous.

The herbaceous and shrub form a thick layer, especially grasses, making it difficult to distinguish individuals in both the layers as woodlands or as herbaceous due to many overhead structures being in accordance with shoots from the same root (Felfili et al., 2002).

The Cerrado *sensu strictu* is characterized by the presence of bent and twisted low trees; the shrub and herbaceous strata exhibits rapid growth during the rainy season (Ribeiro and Walter, 2008). These authors report that the Cerrado species have bent, twisted and gnarled timber trunks, leathery and rigid leaves, as adaptations to the dry environmental conditions. The most common species are represented by the Vochysiaceae and Fabaceae families, as well as species of Malpighiaceae, Anacardiaceae, Salicaceae, Rubiaceae (Felfili et al., 2002, Miranda et al., 2006), among others such as those represented by Caryocaraceae and Annonaceae families (Sales et al., 2009a; Sales et al., 2009b).

In regards climate, the average temperatures in the Cerrado areas vary between 22 ° C and 27 ° C (Klink and Machado, 2005) , with average annual rainfall of 1,500 mm , water deficiency ranging from three to seven months of the year, depending on the region's seasonal (Nimer, 1989). The Cerrado's vegetation occurs predominantly in deep and well drained soil (Reatto et al., 1998), which present a lack of nutrients such as phosphorus and nitrogen , the pH being between 4.5 and 5.5, with high aluminum frequency rates (Ribeiro and Walter, 2008).

Anthelmintic Efficacy of Plant Species from Cerrado for Control of Gastrointestinal Nematodes

In recent years, society has prioritized environmental aspects, directing ample research towards the discovery of new bioactive substances that may be used in integrated pest management, with fewer negative effects on the environment (Castro, 1989).

In an attempt to contribute with an effective alternative control of gastrointestinal nematodes in small ruminants, several researchers have attempted to test plants used in folk medicine, evaluating the efficacy and safety of the same. Plant species rich in tannins called secondary metabolites have been extensively studied. The tannins anthelmintic action may act directly by interfering with the natural cycle of helminths, or indirectly, to protect the protein intake of ruminal degradation (with increased of protein availability in the lower gastrointestinal tract), which complicates the determination of its actual antiparasitic effect (Ketzis et al., 2006).

Furthermore, the results of *in vivo* tests conducted with these forages can be influenced by natural variations in the composition of the plant (by environmental factors or of their own cycle) that alter the concentration of the tannin intake by the animals (Athanasiadou and Kyriazakis, 2004).

The anthelmintic activity, attributed to tannins is present in plant species (Hoste et al., 2006). Calderon-Quintal et al. (2010) suggest that different strains of *H. contortus* show different sensitivities to the extracts rich in tannin and further studies are needed to confirm the *in vivo* results.

Chenopodium ambrosioides L. (Chenopodiaceae) "erva-de-santa-maria", popularly known for its anthelmintic efficacy is a plant of the Chenopodiaceae family, with stem one meter tall with leaves shaped like spears with sinuous edges. The flowers are greenish, clustered in a small bouquet. From the leaves and flowers of this plant may be extracted an essential oil consisting of a mixture of mainly ascaridiol, silvestreno and safrole, and p-cymene and isohametina. The essential oil contains 60-80 % of ascaridiol with proven anthelmintic potential, abundant in the fruit, followed by flowers and leaves (Oliver-Bever, 1983).

Ketzis et al. (2002), working with essential oil of *C. ambrosioides* (0.2 mL/Kg^{-1} of body weight) achieved similar thiabendazole efficacy, promoting the impracticability of all the hatched larvae of *Haemonchus contortus* in sheep. However, Vieira (1992) noted no effect when administered infused orally to cattle.

The Annonaceae family includes about 50 genera and the genus *Annona* being one of the most important. The Annonaceae is characterized mainly by presenting a class of acetogenin substances. These substances are derived from long chain fatty acids, which act as potent inhibitor of mitochondrial respiration (Wang et al., 2002). The biological activities of *Annona* extracts have been attributed to the occurrence of annonaceous acetogenins, a class of natural compounds extracted from leaves (Geum-Soog et al., 1998; Wu et al., 1995) and seeds (Chang and Wu, 2001).

Annona squamosa L. (Annonaceae), known as the Earl fruit, "pinha" or "ata" are trees that can reach up to 5 m in height with long, thin and oval leaves. Its flowers have a greenish yellow color, adapting well to climates with little rain and with a well-defined dry season (Morton, 1987). Amorim et al. (1996) evaluated the aqueous extract from *A. squamosa* leaves, *in vitro*, on the first larval stages of gastrointestinal nematodes of cattle, obtaining mortality of 19.4%. Vieira and Cavalcante (1999) tested *A. squamosa in vivo* on gastrointestinal nematodes in goats. The plant reduced by 40% the count of *H. contortus* eggs in feces. With respect to adult forms of the parasites, *A. squamosa* showed reduction rates in the population of *H. contortus* and *Trichostrongylus columbriformis* of 21.8 % and 31.4 %, respectively, however not reducing the *Strongyloides papillosus* population. Yet according to the authors, the extract showed still to be effective against the adult form of *Oesophagostomum columbianum*, reducing by 74 % the parasites. The acute toxicity of plants from the Annonacea family is still poorly studied and research approaches its *in vitro* cytotoxic efficacy and with possible emphasis on the anti-tumor effects (Vieira and Cavalcante, 1999).

Annona muricata L. (Annonaceae), popularly known as graviola, is a medium -sized fruit tree commonly found in the tropics. The species has been widely used in folk medicine as an anthelmintic, antipyretic, sedative, antispasmodic, and anticonvulsant and as a hypotensive agent in humans (Costa et al., 2002). *In vitro* tests to evaluate the inhibition of egg hatching, larval and adult worm motility are widely used in prospecting for new anthelmintic agents (Vasconcelos et al., 2007).

Ferreira et al. (2013), researching *H. contortus* in sheep, demonstrated that aqueous extract of *A. muricata* leaves at 50, 25, 12.5 and 6.25% concentrations inhibited larval hatching in 84, 9 , 79, 1, 66, 9 and 47.42%, respectively. The authors also evaluated the effect on the motility of L3 *H. contortus* larvae at the same concentrations and obtained reduction motility rates at 83.29%, 89.08 %, 74.62% and 30.47%, indicating significant activity of *A. muricata* on infective larvae of this parasite. However, when were evaluated the activity of the extract on the motility of adult parasites, the response was not dependent on dosage, being able to observe the extracts activity at different concentrations within the first six hours of exposure. Phytochemical analysis did not reveal any type of acetogenins or even alkaloids in the extract but indicated the presence of phenolic compounds in the aqueous leaf extract of *A. muricata* (Ferreira et al., 2013)

Furthermore, since acetogenins have been associated with neurodegeneration in rats and in humans (Champy et al., 2004) the absence of acetogenins in the *A. muricata* extract is a somewhat of a motivating fact, because it can make for this aqueous extract a safe drug to treat targeted animals if compared with plant extracts prepared with organic solvents presuming the extraction of acetogenin (Ferreira et al., 2013).

Annona crassiflora Mart. (Annonacea) commonly known as "panã", "araticum", "cabeça de negro" , "cascudo", "cortiça", "marolo" ou "pinha do cerrado", stands out due to the fruit's flavor, and is used in alternative medicine for possessing antibacterial and antifungal properties (Almeida et al., 1998). It is characterized by being a timber tree species, deciduous in the dry season, hermaphrodite and xerophytic. The phenology of this species is established by flowering early in the rainy season, which occurs from September to December, with fruiting having started in November, with ripened fruit from January to March (Lorenzi and Matos, 2002). The fruits are used as food and appreciated for having a sweet and yellowish pulp with a strong aroma (Roesler et al., 2007).

Queiroz et al. (2012), using ethanol extract from the leaves of *A. crassiflora* verified the action of this extract on *H. contortus* larval development in sheep at 100 and 50 mg/mL^{-1}. The authors also obtained an anthelmintic efficacy superior to 98.6% for the larval development of *H. contortus*, using dried leaves of the same plant at a coproculture concentration of 333.3 mg $(ms)/mL^{-1}$. The aqueous extract from the seeds and leaves of *A. crassiflora* showed anthelmintic efficacy of 99.43 % and 89.81%, respectively at 100 mg/mL^{-1} (Nogueira, 2009), presenting a promising alternative for the control of *H. contortus* in sheep.

In Southeastern region of Brazil, and especially in the North and Northeast, the "cajazeira" (*Spondias mombin* L.) also known as "caja-mirim", "ambaró", "taperebá", is a fruit species belonging to the Anacardiaceae family. Utilized as source of permanent shading for the cocoa tree, it is also utilized by producing fruits that serve as an important source of additional income for the producer. The fruits' juicy, yellow, sour and aromatic properties are appreciated in refreshments and liquors (Sacramento, 2000). The use of the "cajazeira" in folk medicine and by the pharmaceutical industry has increased, being utilized in the treatment of fevers, as an antidiarrheal, antidesintéric, antiblenorrágic and anti-hemorroidiary. According Sacramento (2000), research has recently revealed that the leaf extract contains ellagic tannins giving the plant antiviral properties. Ademola et al. (2005), using the *S. mombin* aqueous and ethanol extract against *H. contortus*, obtained a reduction of approximately 65% of eggs found in the sheep feces (OPG) at a 500 pc mg/Kg^{-1} concentration.

Lippia sidoides Cham. (Verbenaceae) or alecrim pimenta is a species often used as herbal medicine in Northeast of Brazil, due to the antiseptic action owing to the high levels of thymol and carvacrol (Matos and Oliveira, 1998). According Camurça-Vasconcelos et al. (2007) and Vasconcelos (2006), the essential oil of *L. sidoides* possess an inhibitory effect in vitro on *H. contortus* eggs in sheep at 0.02 mg/mL^{-1} to 1.25 mg/mL^{-1}, respectively. Souza et al. (2010), Bevillaqua et al. (2005), and Person (2001), obtained same results using this oil at 0.5% and 1%, respectively. In tests conducted *in vivo*, Camurça-Vasconcelos et al. (2008), reported an efficacy of 54% from the oil of *L. sidoides* in the control of *H. contortus* in sheep at a 283 mg/Kg^{-1}, 14 days after treatment.

The genus *Caryocar*, one of the representatives of the family Caryocaraceae family, has 16 species that are found in South and Central America (Maya et al., 2008). *Caryocar brasiliense* Cambess. specie is a tree species native to the Cerrado regions with wide distribution in the Southeast and Midwest of Brazil (Maia et al., 2008). The popular name of this plant species may vary according to the region of occurrence, the most common being: “Pequi”, “Piqui”, “piquiá-bravo”, “amêndoa de espinho”, “grão de cavalo”, “pequiá”, “pequiá-pedra”, “pequerim”, “Suari”and “piquiá” (Santos et al. 2004). Fruiting is annual and harvesting occurring in the period lasting from September to February (Vera et al., 2005).

The aqueous extract from the *C. brasiliense* fruit peels, at 200 mg/mL^{-1}, significantly inhibited the development of *H. contortus* larvae in sheep. The plant extracts effectiveness in the inhibition of larval development was of 94.8%. The egg-hatching inhibition of LC50 and LC90 was of 23.82 and 53.19 mg/mL^{-1}, respectively. The qualitative phytochemical tests performed in this study indicated the presence of catechins, steroids, flavonoids, saponins, total tannins, xanthones and tannins catechetical (Nery, 2009).

Nogueira et al. (2012) evaluated the aqueous extract of *C. brasiliense* fruit’s skin in the egg hatching inhibition test, with concentrations at 15 and 7.5 mg/mL^{-1}, reported anthelminthic efficacy corresponding to 98.7% and 91.8 %, respectively. For these concentrations, the average L1 were significantly lower than treatment with distilled water or albendazole. The average for unembryonated eggs observed in all the treatments by extract was not different from the distilled water control and suggests that “Pequi” metabolites do not inhibit the embryogenesis of these nematodes, while they may reduce hatching. The egg-hatching inhibition of LC50 and LC90 were 3.81 and 7.35 mg/mL^{-1}, respectively.

In vivo, the average fecal egg count observed for the groups treated with the aqueous extract fruit peels of “Pequi” differed from the untreated group at concentration 2 g/Kg^{-1} bw. During the first and second weeks of post treatment, it was observed a 33 and 32.2% of anthelminthic efficacy *in vivo*, respectively, compared to pretreatment when all animals showed high levels of infection (Nogueira et al., 2012).

The crude powder derived from the "Pequi" fruit peels and leaves showed high efficiency (superior to 90 %) for the inhibition of larval development (LPGF) of *H. contortus* in sheep. The average LPGF for the concentrations at 250, 200 and 150 mg/mL were statistically similar to those observed for the control with the commercial anthelmintic. The aqueous extract from the leaves of the "Pequi" showed higher anthelmintic action within seven days of incubation. The lethal concentrations of LC50 and LC90 after seven days of incubation were 34.95 and 79.74 mg/mL, respectively, for the crude powder of the fruit peels and 69.05 and 97.19 mg/mL for the crude powder from the leaves. For the aqueous extract of the leaves, the LC50 and LC90 were 56.36 and 115.65 and mg/mL^{-1}, respectively (Fonseca, 2012).

Morais-Costa et al. (2012) compared the efficacy of *C. brasiliense* from the northern and central region of Minas Gerais in Brazil. For both regions, the concentration 333.33 mg/mL^{-1} of dried leaves of *C. brasiliense* showed higher efficacy than negative control with distilled water and showed anthelmintic activity similar to the control with ivermectin (16 mg/mL^{-1}). The dried leaves of this plant from northern and central region had anthelmintic action with efficacy of 98.52 % and 83.09 % respectively. This difference could be related to vegetation/area where the species were collected, since the area of vegetation in the northern region is a native and preserved area, which favors better performance and establishment of plant species in the Cerrado.

The species *Anacardium occidentale* L. belonging to the Anacardiaceae family, is popularly known as cashew tree (cajueiro). It is native to Brazil and used in traditional medicine, especially in northeastern Brazil due to its therapeutic effects. In the literature, there are proven pharmacological activities, as the cajueiro being anti-inflammatory plant (Olajide, 2004), ant diabetic (Barbosa-Filho et al., 2005), inhibitor of acetylcholinesterase (Barbosa-Filho et al., 2006) and antimicrobial (Akinpelu, 2001). Aiming to evaluate the anti-parasitic activity of *Anacardium humile* A. St. - Hil. (Anacardiaceae). Nery et al. (2010), used aqueous and ethanolic extracts of leaves against different species of gastrointestinal nematodes in sheep. The aqueous extract anthelmintic activity showed significantly higher than negative control at all concentrations. At concentrations of 150 and 187.5 mg/mL^{-1}, the percent efficacy was not significantly different from ivermectin (positive control, 16 mg/mL^{-1}). The LD50 in the inhibition assay for larval development was 10.14 mg/mL^{-1}, and for the 5% confidence interval it was

13.36-6.83 mg/mL^{-1}. Results of the ethanolic extract were not significantly different from ivermectin at 60 mg/mL^{-1}. The LD50 was mg/mL^{-1} 23.24. Larvae of *Haemonchus* spp. (68%), *Strongyloides* spp. (31%) and *Trichostrogylus* spp. (1%) were identified in the coprocultures of the negative control group. This suggests that the extracts were effective against the three nematodes considered to be the most prevalent and pathogenic in sheep (Ueno and Gonçalves, 1998).

Morais-Costa et al. (2012), in preliminary study, the activity of anthelmintic was evaluated to *Paullinea* sp. on gastrointestinal nematodes of sheep. The leaves of this plant were collected in the city of Montes Claros, Brazil. In this study, *Paullinea* sp. at 333.3 mg/mL^{-1} differed from the treatment with distilled water and showed anthelmintic activity of 70.12 %, similar to treatment with ivermectin. In the control group, 100% of larvae were *Haemonchus* sp. The anthelmintic activity of the Sapindaceae family and the species *Paullinea* sp. may be associated with saponin and tannin respectively.

The "genipapo" (*Genipa americana* L.), Rubiaceae family, tree that has been used in folk medicine, foods and animal feed , leather tanning, forestry, and by logging industries. The species, native to South America, has ecological importance, and is suitable for planting in degraded areas and wetlands (Epistein, 2001). In the egg hatching inhibition test, the aqueous extract of *G. american* leaves at 100 mg/mL, completely inhibited hatching. The relative average number of embryonated eggs was significantly greater than those of unembryonated eggs at 75 and 100 mg/mL^{-1}. This observation suggests a greater efficacy in inhibiting hatching rather than interfering with embryo development. The LC50 and LC90 of aqueous extract from *G. American* leaves were 34.3 and 79.8 mg/mL^{-1}, respectively. In the larval development inhibition test, concentrations $\geq$ 30 mg/mL^{-1} showed anthelminthic efficacy above 94 %. The LC50 and LC90 mg/mL^{-1} were 14.6 and 28.7, respectively (Nery, 2009). This suggests that the extracts were effective against the several nematodes considered to be the most prevalent and pathogenic in sheep (Wood et al., 1995), showing a wide spectrum of action. However, using the hydro-alcoholic extract from the leaves of "genipapo", Krychak-Furtado (2006) found 100% efficacy for EHI at 50 mg/mL^{-1}, thus suggesting the metabolites extracted with alcohol could also show action against nematode eggs.

In an experiment conducted by Costa (2010), the species *Schinopsis brasiliensis* Engl. (Anacardiaceae), *Baccharis tridentata* Vahl. (Asteraceae), *Ximenia americana* L. (Olacaceae), *Lippia sidoides* Cham. (Verbenaceae), *Paullinea* sp. (Sapindaceae) were selected by ruminants in the Cerrado, which are considered to be anthelmintic and tanniferous. The animals showed no worm problems during this research, but there is a need for *in vitro* and *in vivo* to better evaluate the effectiveness of these species.

It was reported by Morais-Costa et al. (2012) at a 333.3 mg/mL, the effectiveness of the dried leaves derived from the plant species *Evolvulus* sp. (Convolvulaceae), *Acosmium dasicarpum (*Vogel) (Fabaceae Faboideae) *Heteropterys byrsonymifolia* A. Juss. (Malphigiaceae), *Lippia sidoides* Cham. (Verbenaceae), *Erytroxylum deciduum* A.St.-Hil. (Erythroxylaceae), *Senna spectabilis* (DC.) HSIrwin & Barneby (Fabaceae), *Baccharis tridentata* Vahl. (Asteraceae), *Casearia sylvestris* Sw (Salicaceae), *Paullinea* sp. (Sapindaceae), *Piptadenia viridiflora* (Kunth) Benth (Fabaceae) and *Ximenia americana* L. (Olacaceae). After the logarithmic transformation and variance analysis, it was found that the average LDPG for treatments with the dehydrated leaves, did not differ from the control by ivermectin, and the efficacies were: *X. Americana* (99.84%), *P. viridiflora* (85.77%), *Paullinea* sp. (70.12%) and *C. sylvestris* (43.63%). This effect can be attributed to condensed tannin concentrations at 10 mg of ethanol extracts from *C. sylvestris* (7.36%) *Paullinea* sp. (6.37%), *P.viridiflora* (1.75%) and *X. Americana* (0.36%). This study demonstrates a potent anthelmintic activity *in vitro*, for the ethanol extract. The fact that some species of this study have low condensed tannin content highlights the synergism among chemical compounds.

Final Considerations

It is necessary to scientifically validate new alternative anthelmintic compounds, characterizing them in the control of ruminant GNIs, and to evaluate the toxicity of these compounds, *in vivo* experiments should be performed, providing some of the plant species to the animals. Thus, species rich in tannins, catechetic tannins, catechins, steroids, flavonoids, xanthones and saponins have promising potential in the control of nematodes of ruminants and furthermore, can be active in synergism of these metabolites.

The species *Anacardium occidentale, Annona crassiflora, A. muricata, A. squamosa, Caryocar brasiliensis, Chenopodium ambrosioides, Genipa americana Lippia sidoides, Paullinea* sp., *Piptadenia viridiflora, Spondias monbin and Ximenia Americana* are adapted to the Cerrado and showed very promising results in reducing the bioactivity in the development of gastrointestinal nematodes of ruminants in Brazil.

In order to clarify the mechanisms of action from extracts of plant species, on the development of larvae using an electronic microscopy, would be a tool to support the study on reducing the use of chemical products, favoring lower incidences of residues in products of animal origin, thereby reducing costs and environmental impacts of these products in the environment.

Plant species rich in tannins, saponins and other secondary compounds, are deserving of further accurate studies to prove the scientific efficacy in controlling gastrointestinal parasites. Therefore, few studies have evaluated the metabolic anthelmintic effect of plant species from the Cerrado as well as possible toxicity effects. Thus, emerges the need to use natural products, based on plant species that are naturally selected by ruminants in this biome.

References

Ademola, IO; Fagbemi, BO; Idowu, SO. Anthelmintis activity of extracts of *Spondias mombin* against gastrointestinal nematodes of sheep: studies in vitro and in vivo. *Tropical Animal Health and Production*, v. 37, n. 3, 223-35, 2005.

Akinpelu, DA. Antimicrobial activity of *Anacardium occidentale* bark. *Fitoterapia*, v. 72, 286-287, 2001.

Almeida, SP. *Frutas nativas do cerrado: caracterização físico-química e fonte potencial de nutrientes*. *In* Cerrado: ambiente e flora. Embrapa-CPAC, Planaltina, 1998, 247-281.

Amarante, AFT; Barbosa, MA; Oliveira, MAG; Carmello, MJ; Padovani, CR. Efeito da administração de oxfendazol, ivermectina e levamisol sobre os exames coproparasitológicos de ovinos. *Brazilian Journal of Veterinary Research and Animal Science*. São Paulo, v. 29, n. 1, 31-38, 1992.

Amorim, A; Rodrigues, MLA; Borba, HR. Influência de extratos vegetais *in vitro* na viabilidade de larvas de nematóides gastrointestinais de bovinos. *Revista Brasileira de Farmácia* , v. 77, 47-48, 1996.

Athanasiadou, S; Kyriazakis, I. Plant secondary metabolites: antiparasitic effects and their role in ruminant production systems. *Proceedings of the Nutrition Society*, v. 63, n. 4, 631-639, 2004.

Athanasiadou, S; Kyriazakis, I; Jackson, F; Coop, RL. Direct anthelmintic effects of condensed tannins towards different gastrointestinal nematodes of sheep: *in vitro* and *in vivo* studies. *Veterirany Parasitology*, v. 99, 205-219. 2001.

Barbosa-Filho, JM; Medeiros, KCP; Diniz, MFFM; Batista, LM; Athayde-Filho, PF; Silva, MS; Da-Cunha, EVL; Almeida, JRGS; Quintans-Júnior, LJ. Natural products inhibitors of the enzyme acetylcholinesterase. *Revista Brasileira de Farmacognosia*, v. 16, 258-285, 2006.

Barbosa-Filho, JM; Vasconcelos, THC; Alencar, AA; Batista, L; Oliveira, RAG; Guedes, DN; Falcão, HS; Moura, MD; Diniz, MFFM; Modesto-Filho, J. Plants and their active constituents from South, Central, and North America with hypoglycemic activity. *Revista Brasileira de Farmacognosia*, v. 15, 392-413, 2005.

Bevilaqua, CML; et al. Ovicidal and larvicidal activity of *Lippia sidoides* and *Ocimum gratissimum* essencial oils against *Haemonchus contortus*. Proceedings oft the 20th International conference of the World Association for the Advancement of Veterinary Parasitology, Christchurch. *New Zealand Veterinary Journal*, v.1, 78-9, 2005. Disponível em: <http//www.sci quest.org.nz.pdf>. Acesso em: 26 agosto 2013.

Bizimenyera, ES; Githiori, JB; Eloff, JN; Swan, GE. In vitro activity of *Peltophorum africanum* Sond. (Fabaceae) extracts on the egg hatching and larval development of the parasitic nematode *Trichostrongylus colubriformis*. *Vet Parasitol*, v. 142, 336-343, 2006.

Calderón-Quintal, JA; Torres-Acostaa, JFJ; Ca Sandoval Castroa, CA; Alonsob, MA; Hoste, H; Aguilar-Caballero, A. Adaptation of *Haemonchus contortus* to condensed tannins: can it be possible? *Arch Med Vet*, v. 42, 165-171, 2010.

Camurça-Vasconcelos, ALF; et al. Anthelmintic activity of *Lippia sidoides* essential oil on sheep gastrointestinal nematodes. *Veterinary Parasitology*, v. 154, 167-70, 2008.

Castro, AG. *Defensivos agrícolas como um fator ecológico*. Jaguariúna. EMBRAPA - CNPDA. Documento, 6, 1989.

Champy, P; Höglinger, GU; Feger, J; Gleye, C; Hocquemiller, R; Laurens, A; Guerineau, V; Laprevote, O; Medja, F; Lombes, A; Michel, PP; Lannuzel, A; Hirsch, EC; Ruberg, M. Annonacin, a lipophilic inhibitor of mitochondrial complex I, induces nigral and striatal neurodegeneration in rats: possible relevance for atypical parkinsonism in Guadeloupe. *J Neurochem*, v. 88, 63-69, 2004.

Chang, FR; Wu, YC. Novel cytotoxic annonaceus acetogenins from *Annona muricata*. *Journal of Natural Products*, v. 64, 925-931, 2001.

Costa, CTC; Morais, SM; Bevilaqua, CML; Souza, MMC; Leite, FKA. Ovicidal effect of *Mangifera indica* L. seeds extracts on *Haemonchus contortus*. *Brazilian Journal of Veterinary Parasitology*, v. 11, 57-60, 2002.

Costa, FM. Influência da estrutura da vegetação na seleção da dieta de ovinos em pastejo, em área de cerrado. Montes Claros, 2010. 78p. Dissertação (Mestrado). Universidade Federal de Minas Gerais/Instituto de Ciências Agrárias, 2010.

Eiten, G. Vegetação do cerrado. In: PINTO, M. N. (Org.). *Cerrado - caracterização, ocupação e perspectivas*. Brasília, DF. Editora da Universidade de Brasília, Brasília, 1993, 17-73.

Epistein, L. Cultivo e aproveitamento do jenipapo. *Rev Bahia Agrícola*, v. 4, 23-24, 2001.

Felfili, JM; Fagg, CW; Silva, JCS; Oliveira, ECL; Pinto, JRR; Silva-Júnior, MC; Ramos, KMO. *Plantas da APA Gama e Cabeça de Veado:* espécies, ecossistemas e recuperação. Brasília: Universidade de Brasília, DF. Departamento de Engenharia Florestal, 2002, 52 p.

Ferreira, LEA; Castro, PMN; Chagas, ACS; França, BSC; Beleboni, ARO. In vitro anthelmintic activity of aqueous leaf extract of *Annona muricata* L. (Annonaceae) against *Haemonchus contortus* from sheep. *Experimental Parasitology*, v. 134, 327-332. 2013.

Fonseca, LD. Potencial anti-helmíntico de *Caryocar brasiliense* Cambess. (Caryocaraceae) no controle de nematódeos gastrintestinais de ruminantes. Montes Claros, 2013. 92p. Dissertação (Mestrado). Universidade Federal de Minas Gerais/Instituto de Ciências Agrárias, 2013.

Fortes, E. *Parasitologia veterinária*. Porto Alegre: Sulina, 606p., 1993.

Geum-Soog, K; Zeng, L; Alali, F; Rogers, LL; Wu, F; Mclaughlin, JL; Sastrodihardjo, S. Two new mono-tetrahydrofuran ring acetogenins, annomuricin E and muricapentocin, from the leaves of Annona muricata. *Journal of Natural Products*, v. 61, 432-436, 1998.

Gopal, RM; Pomroy, WE; West, DM. Resistance of field isolates of *Trichostrongylus colubriformis* and *Ostertagia circumcincta* to ivermectin. International. *Journal for Parasitology*, v. 29, 781-786, 1999.

Hammond, JA; Fielding, D; Bishop, SC. Prospects for plant anthelmintcs in tropical veterinary medicine. *Vet Res Commun*, v. 21, 213-228, 1997.

Hoste, H; Jackson, F; Athanasiadou, S; Thamsborg, SM; Hoskin, SO. The effects of tannin-rich plants on parasitic nematodes in ruminants. *Trends Parasitol.*, v. 22, 253-261, 2006.

Kahn, LP; Diaz-Hernandez, A. *Nutrition: Proceedings of an international conference*. Canberra: Australian Centre for International Agricultural Research. Chapter 5, Tannins with anthelminthic, 2000, 130−139.

Ketzis, JK. et al. Evaluation of efficacy expectations for novel and non-chemical helminth control strategies in ruminants. *Veterinary Parasitology*, v.139, 321-335, 2006.

Ketzis, JK; Taylor, A; Bowman, DD; Brown, DL; Warnick, LD; Erb, HN. *Chenopodium ambrosioides* and its essential oil as treatments for *Haemonchus contortus* and mixed adult-nematode infections in goats. *Small Ruminantes Research*, v. 44, 193-200, 2002.

Klink, CA; Machado, RBA. conservação do cerrado brasileiro. *Megadiversidade*, Belo Horizonte, v. 1, 147-145, 2005.

Krychak-Furtado, S. Alternativas fitoterápicas para o controle da verminose ovina no estado do Paraná: testes in vitro e in vivo. 2006. 147 f. Tese (Doutorado em Agronomia) - Departamento de fitotecnia e fitossanitarismo. Universidade Federal do Paraná, Curitiba, 2006.

Lorenzi, H; Matos, FJA. *Plantas medicinais no Brasil:* nativas e exóticas cultivadas. Nova Odessa: Instituto Plantarum, 2002. v. 2.

Maia, JGS; Andrade, EHA; Silva, MHL. Aroma volatiles of pequi fruit (*Caryocar brasiliense* Camb.). *Journal of Food Composition and Analysis*, v. 21, 574-576, 2008.

Miranda, IS; Almeida, SS; Dantas, PJ. Florística e estrutura de comunidades arbóreas em cerrados de Rondônia, Brasil. *Acta Amazônica*, v. 36, 419-430, 2006.

Mittermeier, N; Myers, RA; Mittermeier, CG. *Hotspots*: earth's biologically richest and most endangered terrestrial ecoregions. Mexico: CEMEX, 1999, 430p.

Molento, MB; Prichard, RK. Effect of multidrug resistance modulators on the activity of ivermectin and moxidectin against selected strains of Haemonchus contortus infective larvae. *Pesq Vet Bras*, v. 21, 117-121, 2001.

Morais-Costa, F; Queiroz, IR; Vasconcelos; Ferreira, AVP; Costa, MAMS; Vieira, TM; Martins, MAD; Duarte, ER; Lima, WS. Efficacy of *Paullinea* sp. (SAPINDACEAE), in the alternative control of gastrointestinal nematodes, Minas Gerais state, Brazil. In: ATBC 2012. Bonito/MS., 2012.

Morais-Costa, F; Cruz, ALMC; Duarte, ER; Lima, WS. Potencial antihelmíntico de espécies vegetais do cerrado, na inibição do desenvolvimento larval de *Haemonchus* spp. In: Encontro de Parasitologia, 2012. Belo Horizonte/MG., 2012.

Morais-Costa, F; Queiroz, IR; Vasconcelos, VO; Fonseca, DL; Ferreira, AVP; Costa, MAMS; Vieira, TM; Mota, GS, Duarte, ER; Lima, WS. Eficácia de Caryocar brasiliense cambess. (Caryocaraceae) de diferentes regiões de minas gerais, no controle alternativo de nematódeos gastrintestinais. In: Congresso de Parasitologia, 2012, São Luiz/MA., 2012.

Morton, JF. Sugar Apple. In: *Fruits of warm climates*, 69-72, 1987.

Nery, PS. Eficácia de extratos vegetais no controle da helmintose ovina, no norte de minas gerais. Montes Claros, 2009. 102p. Dissertação (Mestrado). Universidade Federal de Minas Gerais/Instituto de Ciências Agrárias, 2009.

Nery, PS; Nogueira FA; Martins, ER, Duarte, ER. Effects of *Anacardium humile* leaf extracts on the development of gastrointestinal nematode larvae of sheep. *Veterinary Parasitology*, v.171, 361-364, 2010.

Nimer, E. *Climatologia do Brasil*. Rio de Janeiro: IBGE, 1989, 421 p.

Nogueira, FA, Nery, PS, Ferreira, M; Duarte, ER; Martins, ER. Plantas Medicinais no Controle Alternativo de Verminose em Ovinos. *Rev. Bras. de Agroecologia*, v. 4, n. 2, 2009.

Nogueira, FA; Fonseca, LD; Silva, RB; Ferreira, AVP; Nery, PS; Geraseev, LC; DuartE, ER. In vitro and in vivo efficacy of aqueous extract of *Caryocar brasiliense* Camb. to control gastrointestinal nematodes in sheep *Parasitol Res*, p. 111, 325-330, 2012.

Olajide OA. Effects of *Anacardium occidentale* stem bark extract on in vivo inflammatory models. *Journal of Ethnopharmacology*, v. 95, 139-142, 2004.

Oliver-Bever, B. *Medicinal plants in tropical west Africa. III Anti-infection therapy with higher plants*, v. 9, n. 1, 1983, 1- 85.

Queiroz, IR; Bastos, GA; Ferreira, AVP; Costa, FM; Duarte, ER; Oliveira, NJF. Eficácia de *Annona crasiflora* Mart. (Annonaceae) na inibição do desenvolvimeto larval de nematódeos gastroinstestinais de ovinos. In: XIV Semana da Biologia. 2012. Montes Claros/MG., 2012.

Queiroz, IR; Morais-Costa, F; Vascocelos, VO; Vieira, TM; Fonseca, LD; Ferreira, AVP; Costa, MAMS; Bastos, GA; Duarte, ER; Oliveira, NJFO. uso de *Annona crassiflora* (Annonaceae) no controle de nematóides gastrointestinais de ovinos. In: *Congresso de Parasitologia*. 2012. São Luiz/MA., 2012.

Reatto, A; Correia, JR; Spera, ST. Solos do bioma cerrado. In: SANO, S. M.; ALMEIDA, S. P. (Ed). *Cerrado*: ambiente e flora. Planaltina Embrapa/CPAC, 1998, 47-86.

Ribeiro, JF; Walter, BMT. As principais fitofisionomias do Bioma Cerrado. In: SANO, S. M.; ALMEIDA, S. P.; RIBEIRO, J. F. *Cerrado*: ecologia e flora. Brasília, DF, Embrapa Cerrados, 2008, 279 p.

Sacramento, CK; Souza, FX. de. *Cajá (Spondias mombin L.)*. Jaboticabal: FUNEP, 2000, 42p

Sales, HR; Santos, RM; Nunes, YRF; Morais-Costa, F; Souza, SCA. Caracterização florística de um fragmento de cerrado na APA Estadual do Rio Pandeiros – Bonito de Minas/MG. MG. *Biota*, Belo Horizonte, v. 2, 22-30. 2009.

Sales, HR; Souza, SCA; Luz, GR; Morais-Costa, F; Amaral, VB; Santos, RM; Veloso, MDM; Nunes, YRF. Flora arbórea de uma floresta estacional decidual na APA Estadual do Rio Pandeiros, Januária/MG. MG. *Biota*, Belo Horizonte, v. 2, 31-41, 2009.

Sano, SM; Almeida, SP; Ribeiro, JF. (Org.). *Cerrado*: ecologia e flora. Brasília-DF: Embrapa Informação Tecnológica, 2008, v. 2.

Santos, BR; Paiva, R; Dombroski, JLD; Martinotto, C; Nogueira, RC; Silva, AAN. *Pequizeiro (Caryocar brasiliense Camb.): uma espécie promissora do cerrado brasileiro*. Lavras: Editora Ufla, 2004 (Boletim Técnico).

Silva, GG; Souza, PA; Morais, PLD; Santos, EC; Moura, RD; Menezes, JB. Caracterização do fruto de ameixa silvestre (Ximenia americana L.). *Rev. Bras. Frutic.*, v. 30, 311-314, 2008.

Silva, RB; Rocha, FT; Morão, RP; Nogueira, FA; Marcelo, NA; Duarte, ER. Eficácia de levamizol e albendazol em rebanhos ovinos na região norte de Minas Gerais. In... 47ª Reunião Anual da Sociedade Brasileira de Zootecnia, 2010, Salvador, 2010.

Simões, CMO; Mentz, LA; Schenkel, EP; Irgang, BE; Stehmann, JR. *Plantas da Medicina Popular no Rio Grande do Sul.* Porto Alegre. 5º Edição. Ed. da Universidade/UFRGS, 1998, 42-5.

Souza, WMA; Ramos, RAN; Alves, LC; Coelho, MCOC; Maia, MBS. Avaliação *in vitro* do extrato hidroalcoólico (EHA) de alecrim pimenta (*Lippia sidoides* Cham.) sobre o desenvolvimento de ovos de nematódeos gastrointestinais (Trichostrongylidae). *Revista Brasileira de Plantas Medicinais*, Botucatu, v. 12, 278-281, 2010.

Taylor, MA; Learmount, J; Lunn, E; Morgan, C; Craig, BH. Multipleresistance to anthelmintics in sheep nematodes and comparison of methods used for their detection. *Small Ruminant Res*, p. 86, 67-70, 2009.

Thomaz-Soccol, V; Souza, FP; Cristina Sotomaior, C; Castro, EA; Milczewski, V; Mocelin, G; Pessoa E Silva, MC. Resistance of Gastrointestinal Nematodes to Anthelmintics in Sheep (*Ovis aries*) *Brazilian Archives of Biology and Technology*, v. 47, 41-47, 2004.

Ueno, H; Gonçalves, PC. *Manual para diagnóstico das helmintoses de ruminantes*. Tokyo. Japan International Cooperation Agency, Tokyo, 1998, p. 143.

Vasconcelos, ALC; Bevilaqua, CM; Morais, SM; Maciel, MV; Costa, CT; Macedo, IT; Oliveira, LM; Braga, RR; Silva, RA; Vieira, LS. Anthelmintic activity of *Croton zehntneri* and *Lippia sidoides* essential oils. *Veterinary Parasitology*, v. 148, 288-294, 2007.

Vasconcelos, ALCF. Avaliação da atividade anti-helmíntica dos óleos essenciais de *Lippia sidoides* e *croton zehntneri* sobre nematoides gastrintestinais de ovinos. 2006. 83 f. Tese (Doutorado – Área de Concentração em Reprodução e Sanidade Animal) - Faculdade de Medicina Veterinária, Universidade Estadual do Ceará, Fortaleza, 2006.

Vera, R; Naves, RV; Nascimento, JL; Chaves, LJ; Leandro, WM; Souza, ERB. Caracterização física de frutos do pequizeiro (Caryocar brasiliense Camb.) no estado de Goiás. *Pesquisa Agropecuária Tropical,* v. 35, 71-79, 2005.

Vieira, LS. *Alternativas de Controle da Verminose Gastrintestinal dos Pequenos Ruminantes. EMBRAPA*, 10 p., 2003.

Vieira, LS; et al. Evaluation of anthelmintic efficacy of plants available in Ceará State, North East Brazil, for the control of goat gastrointestinal nematodes. *Revue de Medecine Veterinaire*, Toulouse, v.150, n. 5, 447-452, 1999.

Vieira, LS. *Fitoterapia da Amazônia: manual de plantas medicinais*. São Paulo: Agr. Ceres, 1992, 350 p.

Vieira, LS; Cavalcante, ACR; Pereira MF; Dantas, LB; Ximenes, LJF. Evaluation of anthelmintic efficacy of plants available in Ceará State, North-east Brazil, for the control of goat gastrointestinal nematodes. *Revue Médicine Véterinaire*, v. 150, 447-452, 1999.

Wang, Li-Quan; et al. Annonaceous acetogenins from the leaves of *Annona montana*. *Bioorganic & Medicinal Chemistry*, v.10, 561-565, 2002.

Wood, IB; Amaral, NK; Bairden, K; Duncan, JL; Kassai, T; Malone, JB; Pankavich Jr., JA; Reineche, RK; Slocombe, O; Taylor, SM; Vercruysse, J. World Association for the advancement of veterinary parasitology (W. A. A. V. P.) second edition of guidelines for evaluating the efficacy of anthelmintics in ruminants (bovine, ovine, caprine). *Veterinary Parasitology*, v. 58, 181-213, 1995.

Wolstenholme, AJ; Fairweather, I; Prichard, RK; Von Samson-Himmelstjerna, G; Sangster, NC. Drug resistance in veterinary helminthes. *Trends Parasitol*., v. 20, 469-476, 2004.

Wu, FE; Zeng, L; Gu, ZM; Zhao, GX; Zhang, Y; Schwedler, JT; Mclaughlin, JL; Sastrodihardjo, S; New bioactive monotetrahydrofuran annonaceous acetogenins, annomuricin C and muricatocin C, from the leaves of *Annona muricata*. *Journal of Natural Products*, v. 58, 909-915, 1995.

Zanetti, R. *Análise fitossociológica e alternativas de manejo sustentável da mata da agronomia, Viçosa, Minas Gerais*. Viçosa, UFV. Trabalho integrante do conteúdo programático da disciplina Manejo Sustentado de Florestas Naturais, 1994, 92 p.

In: Anthelmintics
Editor: William Quick
ISBN: 978-1-63117-714-9

Chapter 5

Application of Praziquantel in Experimental Therapy of Larval Cestodoses and Benefits of Combined Therapy and Drug Carriers

Gabriela Hrčkova*[*] *and Samuel Velebný
Department of Experimental Pharmacology, Intitute of Parasitology, Slovak Academy of Sciences, Košice, Slovak Republic

Abstract

Millions of humans and animals are simultaneously infected with different helminth species. However, an important group of disease-causing organisms has often been excluded from such surveys, namely the zoonotic larval cestodoses. In 2007, the World Health Organization included echinococcosis and cysticercosis as a part of a neglected zoonosis subgroup for its strategic plan for the control of neglected tropical diseases (NTDs). Praziquantel (PZQ) has a remarkable range of activity that has been shown to be effective against cestodes and trematodes. It is considered as a drug of choice to control all forms of schistosomiasis in humans and animals. Although it is very well tolerated, and has relatively low level of toxicity and few side effects, much remains to be learned about drug disposition. The very high cost of discovering and developing of new drugs is reflected in the limited number of new classes of antiparasitic agents launched on the market. To identify the new antiparasitic lead compounds, very many compounds will have to be examined in pre-clinical tests. Therefore there is the need of alternative treatment approaches. PZQ has limited water-solubility in biofluids, the result of which is that only a low concentration of the active drug can reach parasites localized in the parenchymal tissues. In this respect, modified drug formulations, which could overcome this problem, can lead to the improvement of efficacy. Spherical lipid vesicles such are liposomes are made from natural lipids and offer many advantages as drug carriers. Immunosuppression of host immune responses, triggered by parasite-derived molecules, is a phenomenon characteristic of helminth infections, and can be manipulated with some drugs (e.g., PZQ) and especially with external immunomodulatory substances. Until a new compound with antiparasitic effect and simultaneous stimulatory activity towards the host´s immunity is available, safe and cheap alternative approaches need to be investigated. There are a numerous compounds isolated from natural sources without having toxic side-effects, which are currently evaluated in antiparasitic therapy, either as single drugs or in combination with current drugs. *Mesocestoides vogae* (syn. *Mesocestoides corti*, Etges, 1991) is considered as a good experimental model to study cestode biology and the effects of drugs, because it can be easily manipulated both *in vivo* and *in vitro* and due to its relatively close relationship with cestodes of medical relevance, such as species of *Echinococcus* or *Taenia*.

The findings summarised in this chapter demonstrate that the efficacy of praziquantel towards larval cestodes can be markedly improved after their incorporation into suitable liposomal drug carriers and application of the immunomodulatory substances, glucan and silymarin offered a very effective tool to activate cells of host immune defence system, which is immunosuppressed towards Th2 response. Finally, our therapeutical approach to combine drugs entrapped in carriers with liposomized glucan or silymarin proved to have multiple advantages over the classical therapy, regarding the efficacy and host pathophysiology.

Introduction

Apart from the free-living turbellarians, the vast majority of species in the phylum Platyhelminthes belong to the three large parasitic lineages of the cestodes (tapeworms), the trematodes (flukes) and the monogeneans (Olson, 2008). Cestodes display some of most fascinating life-cycles of metazoan parasites and some cause serious diseases in humans as well as in animals. Among them, alveolar echinococcosis (AE) caused by *Echinococcus multilocularis*, cystic echinococcosis (CE) caused by *E. granulosus* and cysticercosis, which can be induced by either *Taenia solium* or *T. saginata* are considered the most dangerous for their intermediate hosts, including humans who are infected accidentally.

The genus *Mesocestoides* belongs to the order Cyclophyllidea along with genus *Taenia* and *Echinococcus*, but it is quite unique in several morphologic features seen in adult mature proglottids and a potential three-host life cycle including larval stage called a tetrathyridium (Rausch, 1994; Hrčková et al., 2011). Tetrathyridial larvae were isolated from a large range of small mammals, birds and reptiles, (Specht and Voge, 1965; McAllister et al., 1991; Literák et al., 2004; Zalesny and Hildebrand, 2011). Carnivores (foxes, dogs, coyotes, wolves, etc.) become infected by eating these intermediate hosts, and the adult tapeworms develop in small intestine, releasing gravid proglottids into environment. Tetrathyridia of the species *Mesocestoides corti* were originally isolated from a lizard by Specht and Voge in 1965 and have a unique ability to multiply rapidly by longitudinal anterio-posterior fission in the intermediate hosts, preferentially in the liver and peritoneal cavity, but in experimentally infected Balb/c mice larvae were also found in the mouse mammary glands (Williams and Conn, 1985), lungs and kidney (Todd et al., 1978). This strain was then transferred to several laboratories worldwide and for many years it is in popular use in various experimental studies. *M. corti* was first described in the adult form by Hoeppli (1925) in the house mouse *Mus musculus*, however, no other confirmation of a natural infection in mice harboring adult, strobilar stage exists. Therefore Etges (1991) proposed using the different name for the larval proliferative stage isolated from lizards as *M. vogae*. Due to many biological and molecular similarities with other larval cestode infections and easy maintenance in several laboratory rodents (mice, rats, gerbils), *Mesocestoides vogae* was recommended by WHO (1996) as a suitable model for the slower developing metacestode infections such as *Echinococcus spp.* and *Taenia spp.* in pharmacological, molecular and immunological studies.

A decade ago, the zoonotic larval cestodoses had attracted relatively little attention, although it is estimated that millions people suffer from these diseases at any time, mostly in resource-poor communities worldwide (Vuitton, 2009; Zafar, 2013). In 2007 the World Health Organization included echinococcosis and cysticercosis as a part of a neglected zoonosis subgroup for its strategic plan for the control of neglected tropical diseases (NTDs)

(WHO, 2007). Cystic echinococcosis also known as "hydatid disease" is still a major concern in terms of human and animal infections in South America, North Africa, Central Asia, Western China, Mediterranean basin (Eckert et al., 2001a) and has been imported to Europe and the USA by means of infected animal hosts from endemic countries (Eckert et al., 2001b). Livestock and small ruminants are also at high risk of infection causing significant economic losses, and epidemiological surveys revealed different percentage of prevalence in endemic regions. For example, in northern Italy prevalence of CE ranked between 0.29% (in cattle) and 0.36% (in sheep) (Manfredi et al., 2011).

The highest prevalence of alveolar echinococcsis in humans was reported from poor communities of Western China (3.6%), in Kazakhstan situated in central Asia and in some districts of Russia, particularly in Siberia. This disease occurs sporadically in developed countries on the Northern hemisphere and the annual incidence for example in Western Europe was about 0.5 cases per 100 000 inhabitants. The core endemic area is centered on Switzerland, southern Germany, and eastern France (Torgerson et al., 2010). Over last two decades, red fox populations in Europe have increased as a result of successful rabies vaccination campaigns, which present an increasing risk for humans as well for animals. Infection rate in foxes is high in central Europe where, for example, about 30% prevalence was found in Slovakia (Miterpáková and Dubinský, 2011), 32% in southern Germany (Schelling et al., 1997), 32% in western Switzerland (Brossard et al., 2007) and 35% in Latvia (Bagrade et al., 2008).

Cysticercosis, infection with the larval form of *Taenia solium* (pork tapeworm), is widely prevalent in developing countries of Africa, Asia and Latin America. It is considered by the WHO to be the most common preventable cause of epilepsy in the developing world, with an estimated 2 million people having epilepsy caused by *T. solium* (Coyle et al., 2012). Humans can acquire two different forms of infection – by eating raw or undercooked pork containing *T. solium* cysts (taeniasis), or by eating food contaminated with *T. solium* eggs, (cysticercosis). Localisation of larvae in the central nervous system (CNS) results in neurocysticercosis, which may affect the CNS parenchyma or the cerebrospinal fluid space (Baird et al., 2013). *T. saginata* (beef tapeworm) is a parasite of both cattle and humans causing taeniasis in humans. *T. saginata* occurs where cattle are raised by infected humans maintaining poor hygiene, human feces are improperly disposed of, and where meat is eaten without proper cooking. The highest prevalence of cysticercosis has been reported in Mexico, Central and Latin America, India,

Southeast Asia and sub-Saharan Africa with an estimate of 50 million infected persons worldwide (Kraft, 2007). Rajshekhar et al. (2003) summarized results from seroprevalence studies, which indicated high rates (0.02 – 12.6%) of cysticercosis and range between 0.1 and 6% of taeniosis in several Asian countries (Vietnam, China, Korea and Bali). In European countries prevalence of cysticercosis in animals ranked between 0 to 6.8% (European Commission, 2000). As *T. solium* is not infectious for mice, a related *T. crassiceps* could be used as a reliable model to evaluate therapeutical activity of drugs in vitro and in vivo (Palomares et al., 2004). Infections with other cestode species, either adults or larvae, have been reported in humans as well as animals, often as case reports or sporadic outbreaks. In an immunosuppressed patient infection with *Hymenolepis nana* caused aberrant metastatic larval disease in the liver (Olson et al., 2003) and, interestingly, adult tapeworms identified as belonging to the genus *Mesocestoides* were obtained from a 19-month-old boy in USA, (Fuentes et al., 2003). Human *Mesocestoides* infections were reported also from Japan (Morista et al., 1975; Nagase et al., 1983), Korea (Choi et al., 1967) and China (Fan, 1988), probably having a food-borne origin.

Pathological consequences of these zoonotic cestode infections, mainly in intermediate hosts are severe, associated with tissue damage, granulomatous inflammation, fibrosis, ascites and hypergammaglobulinemia. Moreover, larval tissue of AE and CE possess proliferative capacity and behave as tumors, which can invade neighboring organs. Cells frequently detach from germinal layer of the cysts and disseminate via lymph nodes/ blood vessels, thus leading to the metastasis in a large parenchymatous organs (Craig, 2003). Proliferative tetrathyridia of *Mesocestoides* spp. can be found in dogs and cats, causing severe peritonitis, intestinal ulcerations and infections are often fatal (Crosbie et al., 1998; Toplu et al., 2004; Eleni et al., 2007; Wirtherle et al., 2007; Papini et al., 2010). Among clinical manifestations of human neurocysticercosis (NCC) seizures, epilepsy and severe headache are the most common and most of the pathology is thought to be due to the host immune response to the metacestodes in the brain (Escobar, 1983; Cardona et al., 1999). The crucial role in the overall pathology associated with helminth infections is attributed to characteristic anti-inflammatory Th2–cell and cytokine responses, which is concomitant with impaired cell (T and B) proliferative responses to parasitic and unrelated antigens (Maizels et al., 2004). Immune cells interactions are orchestrated by interleukin 6 (IL-6), IL-9, IL-10, IL-25 and transforming growth factor-β (TGF-β), but the main cytokines are IL-4 and IL-13 (Anthony et al., 2007). The recent advances in understanding the immunoregulatory capabilities of helminth infections revealed that also macrophages are targets for immunoregulation, the result of which is differentiation of alternatively activated macrophages upon exposure to IL-4/IL-13 produced by CD4+ T cells (Reyes and Terrazas, 2007). They play an important role in the protection of the host by decreasing inflammation and promoting tissue repair, however, alternative activation of macrophages also down-regulates host resistance to pathogens (Varin and Gordon, 2009).

Development of new antiparasitic drugs, with different mechanism of activity, is a time consuming and a very costly process. Therefore treatment alternatives are needed to increase the efficacy of anthelmintics, either as drug-drug combinations or co-administration of drug with natural substances. The other possibility of how to increase availability of drugs for tissue parasites is utilization of various carriers and nanoparticles.

Limitation of Monotherapy in Cestodoses

WHO (2007) has identified five drugs (albendazole, diethylcarbamazine-citrate (DEC), ivermectin, mebendazole and praziquantel) in the neglected tropical diseases (NTD) area because they most likely have the greatest and most immediate impact on the public health against a group of helminthiasis. DEC, praziquantel and mebendazole are still not accessible or affordable for poor populations, whereas albendazole and ivermectin are only selectively donated (WHO, 2007). Moreover, praziquantel (PZQ) is drug of choice for the treatment of all *Schistosoma* species (Watson, 2009; EMEA, 1996). In general, PZQ exerts high efficacy against adult stage and schistosomula from age of 6 weeks, however juvenile 4 weeks old schistosomules showed low susceptibility to this drug in vivo (Cioli and Pica-Mattoccia, 2003; Aragon et al., 2009). PZQ acts primarily in the tegument, where induces a Ca^{2+} influx and rise in intra-tegumental calcium leads to increased concentration of Ca^{2+} in the sarcoplasmic reticulum of muscle cells. Disturbance in calcium homeostasis causes immediate and paralytic muscular contractions, followed by death and expulsion of parasites (Mehlhorn et al., 1981). The possible target of this drug, at least in schistosomes, was proposed to be voltage-gated Ca^{2+} channels, which are important regulators of calcium homeostasis in excitable cells (Kohn et al., 2003); however, the precise mechanism of action is still not clear. PZQ is practically insoluble in water, and partially soluble in ethanol and organic solvents. The recommended dose is 40-60 mg/kg body weight (b.w.) depending on parasite species (WHO, 2002). Praziquantel is well absorbed (approximately 80% of the dose) from the gastrointestinal tract.

However, due to extensive first-pass metabolism, only a small part enters the systemic circulation. Praziquantel has a serum half-life of 0.8 – 1.5 hours in adults with normal renal and liver function. In patients with significantly impaired liver function, the serum half-life is increased to 3 – 8 hours. Praziquantel and its metabolites are mainly excreted via the kidney (70 – 80%) within 24 hours after a single oral dose (Steiner et al., 1976; Dayan, 2003). At the standard doses, no toxicity of PZQ was recorded and extensive studies did not show mutagenic potential for humans and it is well tolerated by patients (EMEA, 1996; Montero and Ostrosky, 1997; Olds, 2003).

Most anthelmintic drugs, including benzimidazole carbamates, were developed initially in the response to the considerable market for veterinary anthelmintics in high- and middle-income countries (Geary et al., 2010). Benzimidazoles are used in veterinary medicine as highly effective and safe drugs against nematodes and cestodes (Horton, 1997), which was a prerequisite for the exploitation of their effects in the therapy of human infections. They have proved to be very effective in the treatment of the majority of intestinal infections, however high doses administered for prolonged periods are required for human systemic infections (Dayan, 2003; McManus et al., 2012). Two benzimidazoles, albendazole and mebendazole, are recommended for the therapy of alveolar and cystic echinococcosis (EMEA, 1997; 1999; 2001), alone or prior to and after surgery (Reuter et al., 2000; Vuitton, 2009). Therapy of neurocysticercosis and other forms of human infections with *T. solium* also relies on albendazole due to its principal metabolite, albendazole sulphoxide, but praziquantel is also used (Sotelo and Del Bruto, 2002; Garcia et al., 2002).

The therapeutical potential of PZQ for human and animal cestode infections has been evaluated in many experimental as well clinical studies as single drug regime or in combination, with various level of success. High cestocidal activity was demonstrated against developmental stages residing in the gastro-intestinal tract of the hosts. For example, adult cestodes of *Hymenolepis diminuta* and *H. nana* were completely cleared from their hosts (rats, mice) following a single oral dose of 5 mg/kg and 25 mg/kg of b.w., respectively (Thomas and Gönnert, 1977). Infection with adult tapeworms of *E. multilocularis* in red foxes was nearly completely eradicated following PZQ in bait pellets, which were repeatedly distributed in the natural habitats of foxes during study conducted in southern Germany (Schelling et al., 1997) and France (Roberts and Aubert, 1995). Results provide indirect evidence that the active sites for PZQ activity are present in the tegument of adult tapeworms as well as in protoscoleces of this cestode. In the early study of Taylor and

Morris (1988), the authors showed that praziquantel, at a concentration of 0.01 μg/ml, significantly reduced viability of *E. multilocularis* protoscoleces in vitro and that PZQ was more rapidly effective at much lower concentrations than was albendazole. Similarly, concentrations of PZQ as low as 0.02 μg/ml after 3 h of in vitro incubation had a serious deleterious effect on the ultrastructure of *E. granulosus* protoscoleces (Morris et al., 1986, 1988). In contrast, very little or no effect of PZQ therapy was reported in reduction of *E. multilocularis* cyst growth in intermediate hosts. PZQ treatment of infected cotton rats from 1 month p.i. lasting for a total 6 months with a high daily dose of drug (500 mg/kg b.w.) significantly lowered mass of parasitic tissue. However, 30 days-lasting medication starting 3 months p.i. with daily doses of 100 mg/kg b.w. of PZQ resulted in the higher mean parasite weight than in the control untreated animals (Taylor et al., 1988). Enhanced larval cyst growth of *E. multilocularis* in infected gerbils (*Meriones unguiculatus*) following daily administration of drug (300 mg/kg) between days 29-69 post inoculation was reported also by Marchiondo et al. (1994). Morphological examinations of the cysts from treated animals revealed consistent damage to the ultrastructure and increased blebbings of the germinal membrane into lumen of cysts, what might be responsible for enhanced growth and metastases in the host. In another study on the same experimental model, daily administration 500 ppm of PZQ (0.05% solution) for 35 days reduced parasitic mass by only 12%. These findings suggest that a very high doses of PZQ and prolonged administration are required to induce ultimate damage to the germinal layer, which excluded this drug from being tested in clinical studies for alveolar echinococcosis in animals and humans. Better results were achieved using praziquantel in the therapy of cystic echinococcosis in humans and animals (see for review: Bygott and Chiodini, 2009) in the experimental and clinical studies. The WHO Informal Working Group on Echinococcosis (1996) suggested that PZQ (40 mg/kg) once a week could be added to albendazole therapy, but there are few evidence-based guidelines for its use. For example, in the study of Morris et al. (1990), the effect of PZQ on *E. granulosus* cysts in naturally infected sheep, a model considered to be the closest to the humans, was examined at dose of 50 mg/kg per day given for 6 weeks. After cessation of treatment, at necropsy, one of three sheep had viable cysts and ultrastructural alterations and damage were detected in the cysts from PZQ-treated animals. Outcomes of several clinical studies in patients with CE were not consistent regarding the therapeutical applications. Whilst no effect on the reduction of viability of the liver cysts was seen after two 10-day courses treatment with PZQ (75 mg/kg/day) (Piens et al., 1989), significant killing of protoscoleces (43-64%)

in pulmonary cysts after higher doses of PZQ (210 mg/kg/day) given to patients for 5-6 days were found at the time of surgery (Liu, 1984). In the liver, but not in the lungs, parasitic cysts are surrounded by an "adventitial" fibrous layer formed by the host-derived extracellular matrix components (EMC), what seems to restrict diffusion of drug inside the cysts. In patients with hydatid disease, cyst concentrations of albendazole sulphoxide represented only 22% of serum concentration (Morris et al., 1987), and similar reduced penetration of praziquantel is likely. Administration of PZQ, however, was shown to be highly effective during pre-operative therapy in patients with CE, preventing relapses (Dautovic-Krkic et al., 2002). The main conclusion of the review written by Bygott and Chiodini (2009), and suggestions given by other authors, are that PZQ is not suitable drug in the monotherapy of AE and CE. In addition, PZQ is rather expensive drug for large-scale treatment of animals, like sheep or horses, the exceptions are domestic dogs, cats and other pets. Short-term administration of either PZQ or ABZ to naturally infected dogs with proliferative peritoneal infections caused by metacestodes of *Mesocestoides* spp. was not effective (Crosbie et al., 1998), indicating the necessity to design more effective treatment schedules.

There are only a few reports about the use of PZQ during neurocysticercosis /cysticercosis in humans. Matthaiou et al. (2008) suggested that praziquantel is less effective than albendazole regarding clinically important outcomes after treatment of patients with parenchymal neurocysticercosis. Garcia et al. (2011) showed that better outcomes were achieved after combined therapy with albendazole and praziquantel. *Taenia taeniaeformis* (Cestoda: Taeniidae) has a cosmopolitan geographic distribution. The final hosts are carnivores of the families Felidae, Canidae and Mustelidae, including domestic cats, where worms live in the small intestine. The intermediate hosts of *T. taeniaeformis* are mouse, rat, cat, muskrat, squirrel, rabbit, other rodents, bat and human (Nichol et al., 1981). Treatment options for pet rats infected with *T. taeniaeformis* have not been adequately investigated. However, experimental studies indicate that praziquantel is effective at killing adults and larvae (Eom et al., 1988; Thomas et al., 1982). The safety of praziquantel for the treatment of encysted larvae in rats is unknown, and it is possible that killed larvae would elicit a marked host response that could be harmful to the rats (Irizarry-Rovira et al., 2007).

Combined Therapy with PZQ and Other Drugs

In untreated or insufficiently treated patients with larval infections, recurrence might occur or larvae-associated pathology persists for a very long time. Therefore, great attention is paid to the development of a new treatment schedules and alternative approaches or new drugs with different mechanism of action. A strategy commonly employed in current chemotherapy is the use of combinations of drugs, which enhance efficacy and /or retard the emergence of resistance. Combined chemotherapy is commonly used to control parasitic infections in pets ensuring elimination of different parasitic species. In case of cestode infections, the most studied is combination of albendazole and praziquantel, taking advantage of different mode of action of both anthelmintics on the parasites. Except for AE, a combination of ABZ and PZQ resulted in the higher therapeutical efficacy in many experimental and clinical cestode infections. Several in vitro and in vivo studies revealed that a combination of PZQ with benzimidazole carbamates is a more effective therapeutical alternative for CE as loss of cyst viability and rupture of cysts can be achieved much faster than after monotherapy with ABZ (Morris et al., 1990; Moreno et al., 2001; Urrea-Paris et al., 1999, 2000, 2002). Homeida et al. (1994) evaluated pharmacokinetic behavior of ABZ-sulphoxide and PZQ in men with intestinal parasites showing that co-administration of both drugs resulted in 12-fold increase of ABZ-sulphoxide in plasma when given with PZQ and food, however PZQ pharmacokinetics were not affected, suggesting a synergistic effect.

The combined therapy with simultaneous administration of substances, such as cimetidine, was shown to significantly increase plasma concentration of PZQ in the therapy of neurocysticercosis where a high drug concentration is required (Dachman et al., 1994; Na-Bangchang et al., 1995). Cimetidine can inhibit cytochrome P450 activities, where metabolism of the drug into inactive forms occurs. Jung et al. (1997) showed that its co-administration with PZQ resulted in nearly 100% increase of efficacy in patients suffering from neurocysticercosis. Another potential drug combination for treatment of neurocysticercosis or echinococcosis is praziquantel and albendazole. The cestocidal effect of both, albendazole sulphoxide and PZQ on *T. crassiceps* in mice appeared much earlier than found for each drug given alone. On the ultrastructural level, alterations caused by ABZ and PZQ differed, being more severe after incubation with both drugs (Palomares et al.,

2006). This indicates that a synergistic activity of both drugs on metacestodes could be potentially responsible for the higher efficacy of ABZ (Jiménez-Mejias et al., 2000). Within the last decade, other drug combinations have been evaluated against experimental echinococcosis, for example albendazole with 2-methoxyestradiol, a compound used to interfere with cancer cells proliferation (Spicher et al., 2008).

After decades of mass application of benzimidazole carbamates in the control of gastrointestinal nematodes in livestock, resistant strains have emerged worldwide. Anthelmintic resistance represents threat, which could severely limit current parasite control strategies in humans (Prichard et al., 2012). Mass application of PZQ to control animal infection is limited to carnivores, mostly pets, which decreases selection pressure for the emergence of resistant strains of flatworms. Nevertheless, the risk of developing PZQ resistance exists as the drug is frequently used to control schistosomiasis in humans (Fallon et al., 1995).

Pharmacological Potential of Liposomized Anthelmintics in Experimental Infections

Pharmacologically active compounds are more or less evenly distributed in the whole body and, to reach the target zone, the drug has to cross many other organs, cells, intracellular compartments, etc. where it can be partially inactivated. To overcome this problem, a higher concentration of drug has to be administered, often leading to undesirable side-effects. Once drugs are absorbed into the blood, they are converted to metabolites, which usually achieve peak concentrations within a few hours. Then the elimination of a portion of the parent drug and/or metabolites from the host tissues occurs rapidly. The design of effective therapy is even more complicated if parasites to be killed are localised in the parenchymal tissues, where they are often surrounded by granulomatous inflammatory lesions or collagenous capsules. A possibility of overcoming the problems with a very low absorption of water-insoluble anthelmintics is their entrapment in a suitable carriers (synthetic polymers, liposomes, niosomes, microspheres, nanoparticles, etc.), which can profoundly change the pharmacokinetic behaviour of the drugs (Goyal et al., 2005).

Liposomes are lipid microspheres and, due to their unique structure, they are able to accommodate both lipophilic and hydrophilic substances. Since their preparation by Bangham and colleagues in 1964, they have been used in many fields of biology as non-toxic drug carriers (Gregoriadis, 1977). Data from numerous studies showed that they are versatile drug carriers, which can be used to control retention of entrapped drugs in the presence of biological fluids and controlled vesicle residence in the systemic circulation. In general, liposomes are composed of natural lipids/phospholipids, which are biodegradable, biologically inert, weakly immunogenic, producing no antigenic stimulations and they possess limited intrinsic toxicity. Encouraging results from studies, where drugs entrapped in liposomes were tested for the treatment or prevention of a wide spectrum of diseases in animals and humans, indicate that more liposome-based products for medicinal and veterinary applications could be forthcoming (Allen and Cullis, 2013). These include treatment of skin and eye diseases, antimicrobial and anticancer therapy, vaccines, diagnostic imaging as well as anti-protozoal drug formulations, etc. (Goyal et al., 2005).

To date, very little attention has been given to the research on liposome-based formulations of antiparasitic drugs for humans and the animals (Crommelin et al., 1991; Date et al., 2007). Exceptions are protozoan infections of man: leishmaniasis, trypanosomiasis and malaria, which affect millions of people in tropical and sub-tropical countries. There is expanding number of studies showing that liposomal formulations of anti-protozoan drugs are superior in many ways over the free drugs and several products are already commercially available (Santos-Magalhaes and Mosqueira, 2010). In comparison, there is significantly lower number of studies using liposomal formulations of anthelmintics, although their results are encouraging.

Wen et al. (1996) showed that encapsulation of ABZ into multilamellar liposomes, which were administered to rats with secondary alveolar echinococcosis, increased concentration of albendazole sulphoxide in the liver and plasma. There was a 75-94% reduction in biomass of the metacestode and a significant increase in survival time for the animals treated with liposomized albendazole, which was given in lower doses (35 mg/kg b.w.) than free ABZ at the dose of 50 mg/kg b.w. Similarly, efficacy of liposomized ABZ was higher in comparison with free drug given alone against cysts of *E. granulosus* in experimentally infected mice (Lv et al., 2008) and the antiparasitic effect was enhanced even more after using immunoliposomes with ABZ (Niu et al., 2001). Liposomal formulations of praziquantel proved to be more effective in comparison with free drug in killing trematodes during experimental infections. In the study on *Schistosoma mansoni*-infected mice, Akbarieh et al. (1991) demonstrated that drug concentration of PZQ entrapped in cholesterol-rich multilamellar liposomes given at the dose of 50 mg/kg b.w. persisted in the liver for at least 10 days in comparison with plasma levels after administration of free drug. Using the same experimental model, Mourão et al. (2005) showed that PZQ incorporated in liposomes significantly decreased the load of *Schistosoma* eggs and adults. An increased efficacy of liposome-encapsulated PZQ was observed in the treatment of rats infected with opisthorchiasis, mostly on young liver flukes (Ruenwongsa and Thamavit, 1983). In the study of Shao et al. (1999), liposomized praziquantel (lip.PZQ) was used against the metacestode stage of cystic echinococcosis. The authors demonstrated that lip.PZQ inhibited cyst growth by 68.7%, in comparison with 14.3% inhibition using free PZQ and that the damage to the cysts germinal layer was more severe in the group of mice treated with liposomized drug. During experimental secondary alveolar echinococcosis, a significant increase in inhibition of cyst growth was observed for lip.PZQ in comparison with free PZQ in mice treated with 500 mg/kg b.w. for 12 days for four courses. This seems to be due to the higher concentration of drug in the blood, liver and spleen, which persisted longer after administration. In our studies on experimental infections caused by the proliferative stage of the cestode *Mesocestoides vogae*, deeper insight on the effects of liposomized praziquantel was achieved and summarised in this chapter.

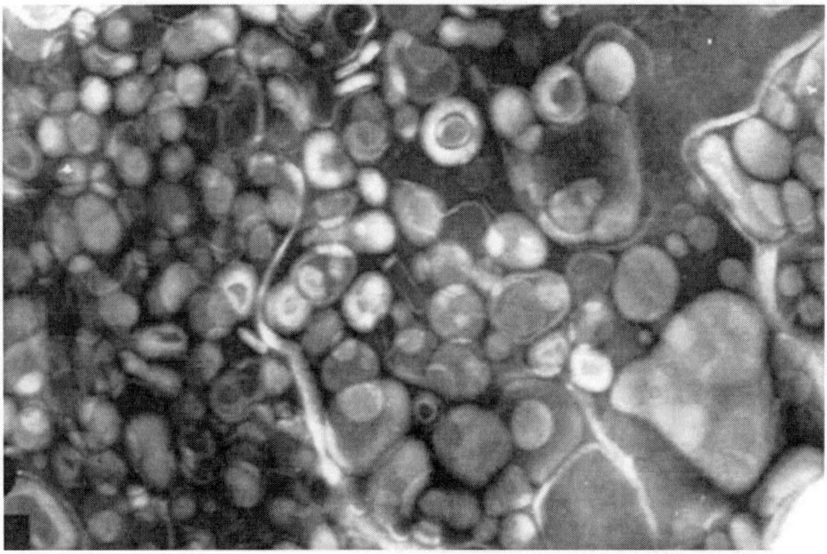

Figure 1. Electron microscopy image of liposomes with incorporated praziquantel.

During the preparation of liposomes, lipophilic drugs such as praziquantel and benzimidazoles are incorporated inside a phosholipid bilayer, together with cholesterol, affecting the physicochemical properties of liposomes. Schepers et al. (1988) showed that PZQ, upon insertion into liposomal membranes, does not modify the lipid structure but acts as a spacer between lipids molecules due to the large area occupied per drug molecule in the lipid layer. We have prepared negatively charged multilamellar liposomes after a modified method (Hrčkova and Velebný, 1995) with (Fig. 1) and without PZQ from dipalmitoyl phosphatidylcholine (DPPC), dicetylphosphate (DCP) and cholesterol (chol), in molar ratio 7:2:1 and the efficiency of PZQ entrapment was 75%. Liposome preparations were characterised by their size-distribution and frequency (%) of the individual size-fractions using a Coulter Counter Model D (Coulter Electronic, UK) showing that incorporation of drug resulted in an overall enlargement of liposome size (Table 1) (Hrčková et al., 2000). As multilamellar liposomes can accommodate higher amount of lipophilic drugs than unilamellar ones, they seem to be suitable carriers for PZQ in the therapy of flatworm infections, and the route of administration is essential for pharmacokinetic behavior of liposomes. In the early work of Thomas and Gönnert (1977), PZQ was effective against tetrathyridia only when administered intraperitoneally in an oily suspension at a dose of 50 mg PZQ, but not after single oral treatment. In our study using ^{3}[H]-cholesterol-labelled liposomes, with and without PZQ (Hrčková et al., 2000), we have shown that after intraperitoneal administration to mice with *M. vogae* infection, they are taken up by peritoneal macrophages which accumulate in the high numbers in the course of infection (Table 2) and monocytes/macrophages in lymphatic system. These cells then release PZQ from liposomes slowly back to the circulation maintaing plasma levels of PZQ for longer period. Hirano and Hunt (1985) demonstrated that the smallest liposomes are usually drained into lymphatic nodes and blood, phagocytosed and transported predominately to the spleen and the liver. It was shown by many authors that cells of MPS can serve as the circulating reservoirs, which leads to the prolonged maintenance and higher availability of unmetabolized PZQ for the parasites in the liver and peritoneal cavity thus increasing the efficacy of treatment. The similar gradual release of albendazole from nanosize liposomes in vitro was reported by Panwar et al. (2010).

Table 1. Size analysis and distribution frequency (%) of individual fractions of [^{3}H]-cholesterol labeled liposomized praziquantel (PZQ) and [^{3}H]-cholesterol labeled liposomes

Size interval of liposomes (μm)	[^{3}H]-liposomes	[^{3}H]-liposomes with PZQ
< 0.8	45.3 %	21.0 %
0.80 – 1.10	9.5 %	10.7 %
1.11 – 1.30	11.5 %	5.6 %
1.31 – 1.60	8.6 %	19.0 %
1.61 – 1.90	9.6 %	14.3 %
1.91 – 2.40	5.5 %	10.0 %
2.41 – 3.00	4.0 %	7.0 %
> 3.01	5.5 %	12.4 %

Legend: The percentage proportion of the liposomal fractions was calculated from the total number of liposome particles counted in 1 μl of the suspensions using a Coulter Counter Model D (Coulter Electronic, UK).

Table 2. In vivo distribution of liposome-incorporated [^{3}H] cholesterol-radioactivity after administration of [^{3}H]-liposomized praziquantel (PZQ) to mice infected with *Mesocestoides vogae* larvae

Examined tissue	Days post infection / proportion of radioactivity (%)				
	1	3	5	8	11
Liver larvae (4mg)	0	0.27±0.03	0.93±0.26	2.18±0.27	9.72±0.70
Peritoneal larvae (4mg)	0.14±0.01	0.17±0.05	0.55±0.07	1.12±0.20	0.38±0.07
Peritoneal cells (2 x 10^7)	8.37±2.08	8.36±0.55	3.07±0.26	3.95±0.44	1.17±0.17
Liver (1g)	2.32±0.42	2.87±0.24	3.15±0.23	1.94±0.19	0.33±0.05
Spleen (1g)	4.68±0.26	2.28±0.17	2.00±0.27	3.25±0.28	3.95±0.33
Abdominal lymph nodes (1g)	0	2.32±0.35	3.97±0.84	1.68±0.13	1.26±0.08

Legend: Data are expressed as proportions of liposome-associated radioactivity (in %) from the total dose (100%) of [^{3}H]-lip.PZQ administered to each mouse.

Values represent the mean ± S.E. (n=8).

Liposomized PZQ was given to mice intraperitoneally in 6 daily doses, (each containing 10 mg/kg b.w. and approximately 40 mg of liposomal lipids), between days 14-19 p.i.

Using the *M. vogae* experimental model and in line with these findings, in the liver the highest efficacy of treatment with 6 daily doses of lip.PZQ (total 60 mg/kg b.w.) was seen on day 7 post therapy (p.t.) in comparison with free PZQ–therapy, which was most effective on day 1 p.t. (Hrčkova and Velebný, 1995). Due to the continuous asexual division of larvae, efficacy of treatment was expressed as their reduction in comparison with untreated control group using the formula:

Percentage of efficacy = 100 x (N control – N treated)/N control
N – number of larvae

The synergistic action of PZQ and the host immune response against *Schistosoma mansoni* was mentioned above and it seems that it also plays an important role in the higher efficacy of liposomized PZQ (lip.PZQ) against tetrathyridia in vivo. Mice infected with *M. vogae* tetrathyridia develop severe hypergammaglobulinaemia (Abraham and Teale, 1987), but immunoglobulins to the somatic antigens associated with larvae seem to protect them from cytotoxic effect of the immune cells (Mitchell et al., 1977). As the result of PZQ action on the tegument, new immunogenic antigens were revealed, which probably triggered production of cytotoxic antibodies. Indeed, more extensive damage to the larval tegument was observed after treatment with lip.PZQ using scanning electron microscopy, in comparison with therapy with free drug (Fig. 2) (Hrčkova et al., 1998). We suppose that due to the sustained presence of drug following therapy with lip.PZQ, groups of larvae showed a greater number of affected worms from the total selected, and characteristic alterations were tegumental lesions, lack of microvilli on the surface of larvae and damage to the deeper layers of tegument. It should be noted that these alterations or damage to tetrathyridia were not uniformly distributed in all of the larvae observed but were rather combined at various intensities. In the *M. vogae* - mouse system, peritoneal macrophages are potential effector cells but their functions seemed to be directly suppressed by tetrathyridia, so as to permit parasite survival (Jenkins et al., 1990, 1991). Recent studies on several helminth model infections revealed that naive macrophages undergo a process of alternative activation upon exposure to parasitic antigens, resulting in down-regulation of nonspecific and specific effector functions. Having in mind the synergistic activity of PZQ with the immune system, the activation of nonspecific effector functions of peritoneal macrophages, namely phagocytosis and the respiratory burst, was examined using the same parasite - mouse model and treatment schedule (Hrčkova and Velebný, 1997). Therapy with lip.PZQ significantly enhanced phagocytic activity (PA) of peritoneal macrophages in vitro, in comparison with untreated mice. When lip.PZQ was administered to mice, PA reached the peak on day 6 p.t., but in groups treated with the same doses of free PZQ, PA peaked earlier, on day 3 p.t., and was lower. The resulting differences could be explained by the different pharmacokinetic behavior of both drug formulations. Administration of lip.PZQ also significantly increased the levels of extracellular superoxide anions produced by macrophages, immediately after the last dose, and this process was only slightly elevated after PZQ therapy.

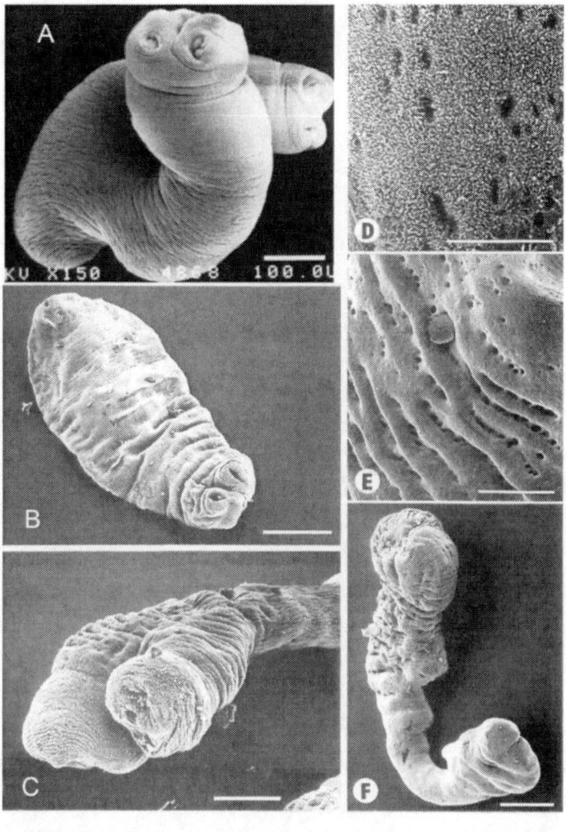

Figure 2. Scanning electron micrographs of the *Mesocestoides vogae* larvae (tetrathyridia) obtained from the peritoneal cavity of infected control mice and after termination of therapy with 6 doses of PZQ or lip.PZQ between days 15-20. Scale bars on individual immages correspond to 100 μm. (A), intact dividing larva from control-untreted mice. (B), moderately flattened and elongated larval body after PZQ administration on day 1 p.t. (C), detail of the anterior part of elongated larva after lip.PZQ therapy on day 5 p.t. (D), surface of the larvae after either treatment showing area lacking microvilli. (E), tegumental "holes" lacking microvilli were deeper after lip.PZQ therapy, on the larvae obtained on day 3 and 5 p.t. (F), an example of larvae from both PZQ-treated mice showing damage to the anterior part of the body in the form of lesions and protuberances. In general, tegumental damage was observed predominately in head and neck regions of the larvae.

We suppose that in the case of lip.PZQ, significant activation of cell effector functions might be triggered following uptake of opsonized liposomes via macrophage surface receptors. We also showed that incubation of PZQ with macrophages in vitro did not trigger a respiratory burst, indicating that the effect of drug is more likely to be indirect, as there are no reports on immunoadjuvant properties of PZQ itself. Alanine aminotransferase (ALT) and aspartate aminotransferase (AST) enzymes are released from liver hepatocytes into blood after the cell damage, which is very intensive during parasitisation and/or migration of helminth larvae/eggs. Administration of free PZQ caused the rapid and pronounced decrease of elevated ALT and AST activities in the serum whereas, after the same dose of PZQ given in liposomes, decline was gradual and lower levels of enzymes persisted for a much longer period p.t. (Velebný and Hrčkova, 1995). Different dynamics of serum levels of liver enzymes fits well with our hypothesis about altered pharmacokinetics of PZQ in liposomes, which seems to be the main factor influencing the efficacy of treatment.

Immunomodulatory Compounds in Combined Therapy with Anthelmintics

It has been demonstrated in many studies, that soluble E/S antigens from cestodes contain higher amounts of carbohydrates than proteins and these glycan molecules are involved in immunoregulation towards to the chronic granulomatous inflammation. Glycoconjugates present in secreted helminth antigens have been proposed to act on immune cells which shift adaptive response towards Th2 type and early interactions are crucial for the outcome of the final immune response (Maizels et al., 2004). In *Echinococcus* spp. infections, at the metacestode stage, studies of the immune responses in the experimental murine model, as well as in humans, have shown that cellular immunity induced by a Th1 type cytokine secretion was able to successfully kill metacestodes at the initial stage of development (Vuitton, 2003). Rigano et al. (2004) referred that T cell lines isolated from the patients with inactive cysts of *E. granulosus* had a Th1 profile, because they exclusively produced IFN-γ, providing in vitro evidence that Th1 lymphocytes contribute decisively to the infection progress. It was documented that, during larval cestode infections, a shift towards Th2 type response is associated with highly suppressed secretion of IFN-γ. Therefore, combined therapy with an anthelmintic and a compound which would be able to activate the pro-inflammatory arms of the immune system seems to be a possible treatment alternative.

In agreement, more effective therapy of experimental alveolar echinococcosis in mice with albendazole in combination with transfer factor (Dvorožňaková et al., 2009) or with liposomized muramyltripeptide phosphatidylethanolamine (Dvorožňaková et al., 2008) induced long-term development of protective Th1 response, with significantly increased serum levels of IFN-γ and decreased concentration of IL-5.

Glucan in Therapy of Experimental Metacestode Infections

Glucans are (1-3)-β-D-linked polymers of glucose found in the cell walls of fungi, bacteria, yeast and several plants, and belong to a class of drugs known as biological response modifiers. They can non-specifically activate innate immunity cells (monocytes/macrophages, dendritic cells, neutrophils and NK cells) upon binding to the group of specific receptors called "pattern recognition receptors", namely dectin-1 on macrophages and neutrophils, CR3 receptors (Taylor et al., 2002; Herre et al., 2004) and monocyte scavenger receptors (Rice et al., 2002). Binding of glucans to these receptors triggers a cascade of events resulting in the expression of pro-inflammatory cytokines, predominately TNF-α as well as cytokines IL-1, IL-2 and IL-6 (Williams et al., 2000; Majtán et al., 2005; Vetvička et al., 1996). Recently, Chen et al. (2013) reported that β-(1-3)-glucan from fungi affects the balance of Th1/Th2 cytokines by promoting secretion of anti-inflammatory cytokines in vitro and Municio et al. (2013) stated that response of human macrophages to β-glucans depends on the inflammatory milieu.

Results from the studies on various infection diseases indicated the beneficial effect of glucan alone, or in combination with drugs, in the therapy. During experimental toxocariasis in mice, a striking reduction in numbers of *T. canis* larvae in muscles was observed after administration of β-glucan alone (Šoltýs et al., 1996) and larval killing was even more effective after combined therapy with soluble β-glucan and benzimidazole carbamates entrapped in liposomes (Hrčkova and Velebný, 2000). Another type of β-glucan, isolated from oat, was able to enhance resistance to the protozoan parasite *Eimeria vermiformis* in immunosuppressed mice and to stimulate proliferation of INF-γ as well as IL-4 secreting cells (Yun et al., 1997). In sheep infected naturally with gastrointestinal nematodes, administration of albendazole in combination with β-glucan improved efficacy and resulted in significant reduction in egg outputs within the period of 3 months p.t., more than did therapy with a single drug (Várady et al., 2005).

In a series of our studies, we examined for the first time the effects of combined therapy with free or liposomized glucan and/or the anthelmintic drug praziquantel using the *Mesocestoides vogae*-mouse model. A soluble form of β-(1-3)-D glucan, isolated from *Saccharomyces cerevisiae* (MEVAK, Slovak Republic), was obtained after carboxymethylation (Kogan et al., 1988). Nine doses of this CM-glucan, each comprising 5mg/kg b.w. either free or entrapped in water compartments of negatively-charged liposomes, were given subcutaneously to infected mice, and both treatments resulted in a significant reduction of larval counts (Ditteová et al., 2003). However, in the liver, this was accompanied with more intense fibrosis determined by means of hydroxyproline concentration.

In the case of administration of liposomized glucan (lip.Glu), lecitin from liposomes contributed to the partial reparation of parenchymal liver cells indicated by lower ALT and AST serum levels. When testing dose-dependent effect of CM-glucan on this model, we have found a negative correlation between larval burden and fibrosis (Ditteová et al., 2005). So the highest dosage of glucan administered in vivo resulted in the highest intensity of fibrosis. In agreement with our data, therapeutical administration of multiple doses of the polysaccharide lentinan, to mice infected with tetrathyridia of *Mesocestoides corti,* markedly decreased larval counts in the peritoneal cavity due to activation of immunity. In the liver, granulomas were larger than in the control and there was more collagen deposition and fibrosis (White et al., 1988).

Hepatic fibrosis is a serious pathological consequence of human echinococcosis, schistosomiasis and infections with other helminths with temporary or long-lasting residence in the liver. In general, it is a host-protecting reaction orchestrated by several immune and liver cells and secreted factors (Friedman, 2000). In alveolar echinococcosis, resistance/susceptibility to larval growth was associated with deposition of EMC around the parasites and fibrosis was more intense in *E. multilocularis* resistant NMRI mice (Guerret et al., 1998) indicating a role in reducing metacestode growth.

In our experiments on *M. vogae* infection, more intense fibrosis was found after termination of therapy with PZQ (total dosage of 210 mg/kg b.w. in 6 doses twice a day) alone and with PZQ in combination with lip.Glu (total 15 mg/kg b.w. in 3 daily doses), in comparison with untreated mice, which correlated with the highest reduction of larval counts (Hrčkova et al., 2006).

Elevated mastocytosis, observed in infected livers, was modulated following therapy, being the most intense after administration of lip.Glu alone (Fig. 3). It has been shown that mast cells secrete various mediators which promote fibroblast growth and production of extracellular matrix components (Monroe et al., 1988; Puxeddu, 2003).

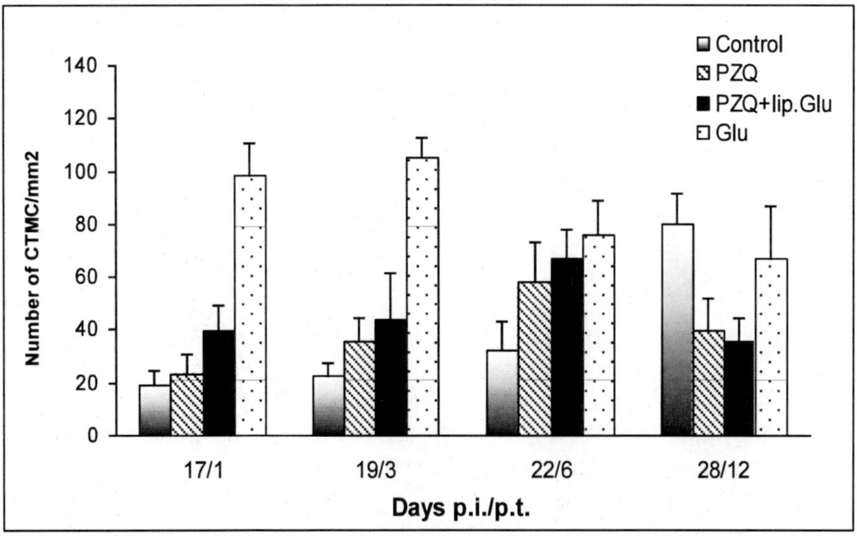

Figure 3. The numbers of connective tisse mast cells (CTMC) present on the liver sections from mice infected with *Mesocestoides vogae* larvae (control) and infected mice during follow-up therapy with praziquantel (PZQ) alone, or in combination with liposomized glucan (lip.Glu) or lip.Glu alone. PZQ was given in 6 doses twice a day (total dose was 60 mg/kg b.w.) between days 14-16 p.i. Lip.Glu was given in 3 doses once a day (total dose was 15 mg/kg b.w.) between days 14-16 p.i. CTMC were stained with toluidine blue solution and cells were counted in the whole area of 80 independent ocular grids at magnification 600x (area of the circle= 0.076 mm^2) and mean mast cell numbers /field were calculated. Figure shows the mean numbers of CTMC for 1mm^2 of the section area for each group of mice.

The presence of a glucan receptor on dermal fibroblasts and the binding of β-glucan suggest that it can also directly stimulate collagen type I and III biosynthesis (Wei et al., 2002). We showed that the glucan´s strong profibrotic activity can be abolished after co-administration of praziquantel, whereas its stimulating effect on macrophage capacity to phagocytose unopsonized particles (1.2 μm) was not affected (Table 3).

Table 3. Phagocytic activity of peritoneal macrophages from mice infected with the tetrathyridia of *Mesocestoides vogae* and treated with PZQ alone or in combination with glucan entrapped in liposomes

Days p.i/ p.t	Experimental groups of mice		
	Control	PZQ	PZQ+lip.Glu
17/ 1	71,5±3.5	75,6 ± 4,0	82,6 ± 3,7*
19 / 3	68,2 ± 2,5	72,3 ± 2,8	78,5 ± 2,1*
22 / 6	65,3 ± 1,9	69,3 ± 3,4	69,1 ± 3,3
28 / 12	61,9 ± 2,4	66,8 ± 2,3	67,8 ± 2,7

Legend: * Significantly lower value in comparison with control-untreated group, (P < 0.05). Data are expressed as the mean ± SD, (n=4).

PZQ was given in 6 doses twice a day (total dose was 60 mg/kg b.w.) between days 14-16.

Lip.glucan was given in 3 doses once a day (total dose was 15 mg/kg b.w.) between days 14-16 p.i.

Phagocytic activity was calculated as proportion (%) of cells containing 3 and more HEMA particles from each 100 counted cells, in total 400 cells were counted for each group.

Phagocytosis is usually accompanied with the respiratory burst in macrophages and neutrophils, the result of which is production of an elevated amount of reactive oxygen species (ROS). In vitro co-incubation of soluble glucan with murine J774 cell line markedly increased free radical levels (Tsiapali et al. 2001) and a similar stimulation of the respiratory burst and microbicidal activity also occurs in eosinophils and neutrophils. Production of superoxide anions by peritoneal macrophages was significantly stimulated following administration of multiple doses of CM-glucan to mice with both *M. vogae* and *E. multilocularis* infections (Porubcová et al., 2007). In the later model, synthesis of IFN-γ and IL-5 decreased after glucan administration, whereas combined therapy with glucan and albendazole resulted in the elevated serum levels of IFN-γ only, along with the highest efficacy of treatment. It has been mentioned previously that PZQ acts on some parasitic flatworms in synergy with antibodies to newly retrieved tegumental antigens. In our study, using infection with tetrathyridia of *M. vogae* (Hrčkova et al., 1997), we showed that administration of PZQ alone and in combination with lip.glucan resulted in marked changes in the dynamics of IgG and IgM antibodies to the somatic larval antigens, which were probably induced by the newly exposed antigens. Moreover, the number of immunogenic larval antigens (analyzed by Western blot) was higher after combined therapy in comparison with single drug administration, which correlated with the intensity of reduction of the larval counts in the liver and peritoneal cavity of mice.

Summarising our data and of others about the effects of β-glucans in several helminth infections, we can conclude that simultaneous administration of smaller doses of soluble β-(1-3)-D glucan with either praziquantel or albendazole leads not only to a significantly increased efficacy but also induces pro-inflammatory changes in innate immunity cells and T and B lymphocytes. In contrast to the profibrotic effect of PZQ and glucan given alone, combined therapy reduced pathophysiological processes such mastocytosis and liver fibrosis, probably by a multistep process, in which mutual interactions with different immune cells were involved.

The Flavonoid Silymarin in Therapy

Flavonoids are plant pigments present in almost all terrestrial plants, where they provide UV protection and color. Although toxicity of most isolated flavonoids to animal cells is very low (Middleton et al., 2000), several ubiquitous flavonoids genistein, curcumin, kaemferol, rutin, quercetin, etc. showed direct toxic effects on various species of helminths (see for review: Hrčkova and Velebný) as well as profound anticancer activity (Zheng et al., 2011; Zhong et al., 2006 and others). However, to date, only a few chemically defined flavonoids and polyphenols have been examined on experimental parasitic flatworm infections alone, or as adjunct to therapy with anthelmintics. Polyphenol paeoniflorin is one of the major constituents of plant *Paeonia lactiflora* Pall., known from ethnomedicine reports. The direct toxic effect of purified paeoniflorin on flatworms has not been demonstrated but its co-administration with praziquantel proved to be superior over the therapy with single drug in experimental infection with *Schistosoma mansoni* (Chu et al., 2007; Chu et al., 2011).

Silymarin (SIL) is a unique flavonoid complex containing silybinin, silydianin and silychristin, which is isolated from seeds of milk thistle, *Silybum marianum* L. Gaertn., and was used as very potent hepato-protective compound in ancient Greek remedies. Its beneficial properties and medicinal applications have been subjects of many studies, which showed its strong antioxidant, anti-mutagenic and anti-cancer activity (Havsteen, 2002). In the last few years, the relevance of the antioxidant and hepatoprotective effect of SIL in the therapy of liver-associated flatworm infections has been demonstrated on the *Schistosoma mansoni*-mouse model (El-Lakkany et al.,

2012) and in our studies on the *Mesocestoides vogae* – mouse model. Migration and multiplication of larvae cause severe damage to the liver parenchyma, which results in oxidative stress, hepatocyte dysfunction, severe inflammation and progression of fibrogenesis. The activation of fibrogenesis is a complex process involving interactions of hepatic stellate cells with hepatocytes, endothelial cells, Kupffer cells and inflammatory cells and is mediated by various cytokines and reactive oxygen species (ROS) (Reeves and Friedman, 2002). Eosinophils, neutrophils and macrophages are ROS producing cells and can be easily localized in the frozen tissue sections. In the livers of mice with *M. vogae* infection they accumulated in the site of injury and around larvae (Fig. 4), where they probably contributed to the activation of hepatic stellate cells by means of high amounts of released ROS.

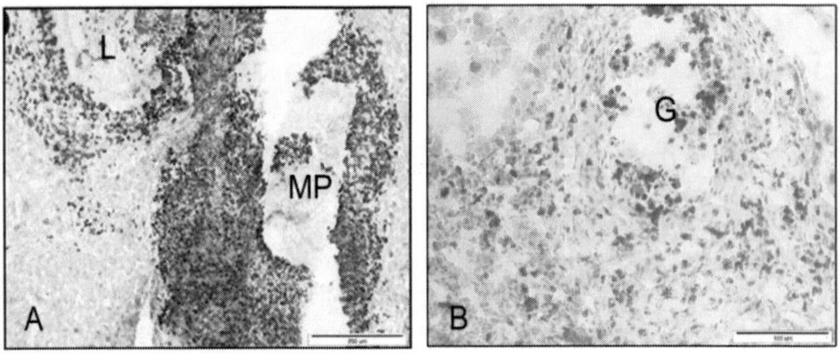

Figure 4. (A, B): Light microscopy images of the liver sections showing acute (A) and chronic (B) inflammatory lesions after the infection with *Mesocestoides vogae* larvae. Granulocytes and macrophages were localized in the frozen sections following binding of substrate DAB (3,3′-Diaminobenzidine) with enzyme peroxidase, involved in the production of reactive oxygen species by these cells. (L-larva, MP- migratory path, G-granuloma).

In our experiments, ten doses of PZQ and SIL (one dose contained 35 mg/kg of PZQ and 30 mg/kg SIL) were given orally between days 15–24 p.i. and efficacy of treatment (%) in the liver after therapy with PZQ alone and in combination with SIL was evaluated from reduction of larvae encapsulated in fibrous tissue and non-encapsulated larvae (Table 4). Co-administration of SIL with PZQ significantly increased efficacy of drug given alone. In both treated groups, non-encapsulated larvae were more susceptible to the therapy, however co-administration of SIL significantly potentiated efficacy also against encapsulated larvae. In vitro incubation of larvae with up to 0.3 mg /ml of SIL (0.2%/ml DMSO) for 72 hours has not adversely affected the viability of larvae and did not cause gross morphological changes, in contrast to the action of PZQ in concentrations as low as 0.3 μg/ml medium (Fig. 5). To explain the significant elevation of efficacy, in spite of the lack of direct toxicity of SIL for larvae, we have performed further experiments. Analyzing many reports dealing with SIL action in vivo and in vitro, we and others suppose that possibly the unifying mechanism is related to early scavenging and antioxidant activity on ROS-induced oxidative stress.

Table 4. Numbers of *Mesocestoides vogae* larvae isolated from the livers of control-untreated mice and treated with praziquantel alone or in combination with silymarin during follow-up therapy

Days	Control		PZQ		PZQ + Silymarin	
p.i./p.t.	non-encapsulated	encapsulated	non-encapsulated	encapsulated	non-encapsulated	encapsulated
25/1	305±49	93±18	188±32*	87±15	143±27*	50±17*
28/4	422±435	256±30	297±50*	136±20*	281±38*	115±31*
35/11	730±73	745±43	560±41*	469±37*	469±40*	227±37*
44/20	808±65	1261±105	875±64	685±51*	788±73	343±56*

Legend:Non-encapsulated larvae were isolated after trypsin digestion and larvae encapsulated in fibrous material were isolated after collagenase type I digestion.

* Significant difference between the larval numbers in the control and treated groups, ($P < 0.05$). Larval counts represent means±SD from two experiments (n=10).

Decreased production of superoxide anions by peritoneal adherent cells determined in our experiments in vitro, and after combined therapy with PZQ and SIL in vivo, has supported this hypothesis (Velebný et al., 2010). There are several enzymatic and non-enzymatic systems responsible for maintaining physiological levels of ROS, among which glutathione (GSH) is most important non-enzymatic antioxidant and redox regulator (Yuan and Kaplowitz, 2009). The key role of hepatic stellate cells (HSC) in the initiation of fibrogenesis is well known and was mentioned earlier. Oxidative stress in tissues contributes to HSC activation indirectly by releasing profibrogenic factors, mainly TGF-β, and also directly by excess of ROS produces by Kupffer cells, neutrophils and eosinophils recruited to the site of injury (Baroni et al., 1998; De Blesser et al., 1999). We have shown that administration of PZQ temporarily decreased GSH levels but did not reduce ROS – stimulated fibrogenesis. Silymarin, by virtue of its direct antioxidant capacity and down-regulation of ROS-production by inflammatory cells, significantly prevented lipid peroxidation, and stimulated GSH synthesis more than was found in uninfected mice.

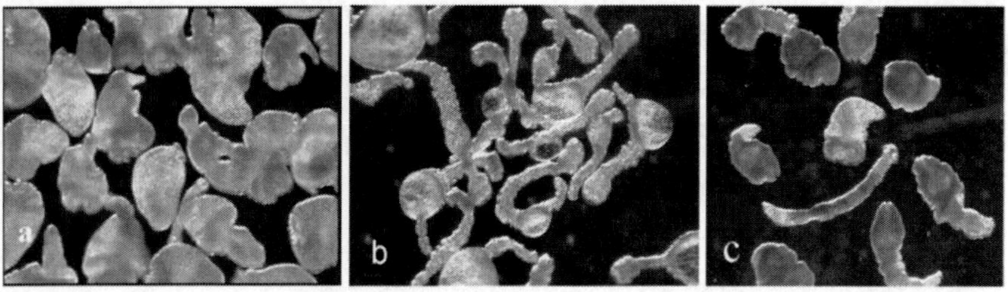

Figure 5. (a-c): Images of *Mesocestoides vogae* larvae in culture flasks following incubation in M199 medium in vitro at 37°C. (a), larvae without any treatment after 72 hours of incubation. (b), dead larvae after 24 hours of incubation with 0.3 μg of PZQ/ml showing body extension and loss of gross morphology due to influx of calcium from medium. (c), viable and highly motile larvae after 72 hours of incubation with 0.3 mg/ml of silymarin.

A very potent antifibrotic effect of SIL in the livers of mice, following combined therapy with PZQ, was another observation consistent with other reports. Suppressed fibrogenesis was reflected by significantly decreased serum levels of hyaluronic acid (HA) (Velebný et al., 2008), which plays a prominent role in the pathogenesis of liver fibrosis and is released into serum from activated hepatic stellate cells (Wu and Zern, 2000). In the liver, a marked decline in hydroxyproline concentration (HP) was observed after combined therapy but not in the group of mice treated with PZQ alone (Table 5). Administration of silymarin alone to infected mice resulted in elevated number of larvae and suppressed fibrosis in the liver (not shown), indirectly supporting the protective role of fibrous material against larval migration and proliferation. In agreement with antifibrotic effect of SIL and tight association between fibrosis and mastocytosis, we have also observed a rapid decline of numbers of connective tissue mast cells (Fig. 6) We have examined further which of two main constituents of extracellular matrix components, namely collagen type I and III, were lowered on the transcriptional level during follow–up therapy. In the PZQ-treated group, elevated HP concentration correlated with moderately increased gene expression of both types of collagens within a week post-treatment, in comparison with untreated controls. Strong antifibrotic activity of SIL has been demonstrated by marked down-regulation of gene expression over a two week period (Fig. 7). In addition, we also demonstrated that administration of silymarin+PZQ, but not PZQ treatment alone, significantly stimulated the proliferation of liver parenchymal cells following nuclear marker bromodeoxyuridine (BrdU) application in vivo. On the contrary, proliferation of profibrotic cells was limited (Velebný et al., 2010). The regulatory role of SIL in cellular processes has been shown to start at the transcriptional level via nuclear factor - κB, (Gharagozloo et al., 2010), which is involved in the regulation of tissue damage and cellular proliferation, as well as inflammatory reactions.

Table 5. Concentration of hydroxyproline (HP) in the livers of mice infected with *Mesocestoides vogae* larvae, untreated (control) and treated with praziquantel (PZQ) alone and in combination with flavonoid silymarin (SIL)

Days	Hydroxyproline concentration (μg/g) in the livers of mice		
p.i./p.t.	Control	PZQ	PZQ + SIL
25/1	279.6 ± 13.7	318.4 ± 11.7♦	185.4 ± 12.5*
28/4	355.7 ± 25.7	385.1 ± 10.4	219.1 ± 13.6*
35/11	417.5 ± 20.2	441.3 ± 18.6	286.3 ± 18.4*
44/20	541.3 ± 28.8	549.2 ± 22.7	429.5 ± 24.6*

Legend: Concentration of HP in the liver of uninfected mice was 76.4 ± 5.8, on day 7 p.i. = 110.4 ± 10.2, on day 14 p.i. = 160.1 ± 18.4, on day 21 p.i. = 242.5 ± 17.8.

* Significantly lower values of HP in comparison with values in control group in corresponding days post therapy, ($P < 0.01$).

♦ Significantly higher value in PZQ-treated group in comparison with the control group on day 1 post therapy, ($P < 0.05$).

Each value represents mean ± SD (n = 10), post infection (p.i.), post therapy (p.t.).

In the light of present data, we believe that in the liver SIL potentiated the larvicidal effect of PZQ indirectly via suppression of oxidative stress and normalisation of GSH redox balance. Elimination of ROS and ROS-induced activation of HSC was down-regulated resulting in decreased collagen synthesis and larval encapsulation. Our in vitro study showed that the free larvae are very susceptible to the drug action. Indeed, lower numbers of both non-encapsulated and encapsulated larvae were found after combined therapy, in contrast with PZQ-therapy, supporting our hypothesis.

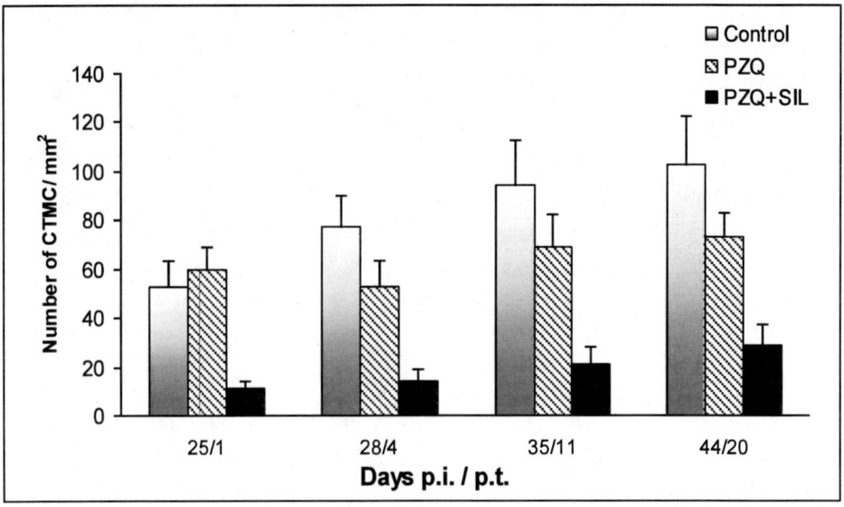

Figure 6. The numbers of connective tissue mast cells (CTMC) present on the liver sections from mice infected with *Mesocestoides vogae* larvae (control) and infected mice during follow-up therapy with praziquantel (PZQ) alone, or in combination with silymarin. PZQ and silymarin were administered to mice in 10 daily doses (total dose of PZQ was 350 mg/kg b.w. and total dose of SIL was 300 mg/kg b.w.) between days 15-24 p.i.

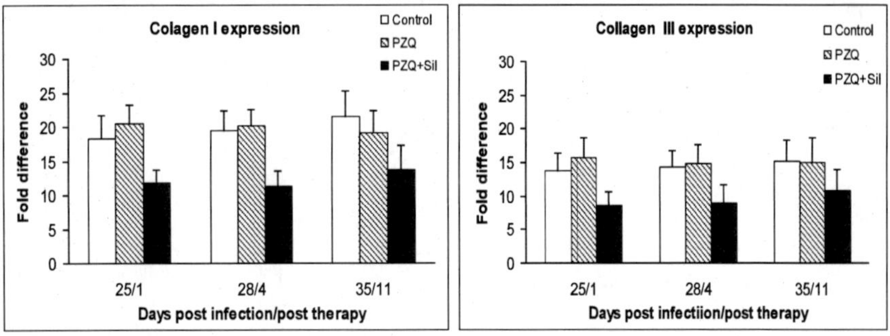

Figure 7. Gene expression profiles measured by real-time PCR of transcribed m-RNAs encoding collagen type I and collagen type III proteins in the livers of infected mice and in mice treated with PZQ alone or in combination with SIL. Total RNA was isolated from the large liver lobes of five mice with *Mesocestoides vogae* infection and 3 μg were reverse transcribed. Results are expressed as the relative gene expression (RGE) value (mean ± SD, n = 5) after comparison with uninfected liver following normalization with β-actin.

After ingestion, larvae of *M. vogae* migrate simultaneously to liver and peritoneal cavity of intermediate hosts where their multiplication is unlimited. Peritonitis caused by proliferative *Mesocestoides* tetrathyria was described also in dogs and cats (Crosbie et al., 1998; Toplu et al., 2004; Eleni et al., 2007; Wirtherle et al., 2007; Papini et al., 2010), with poor prognosis and complicated therapy. Therefore, we were interested whether silymarin can potentiate effect of praziquantel on the larvae in the peritoneal cavity and how treatments modulate the functional state of inflammatory cells. Previous reports showed that peritoneal infection with *M. vogae* larvae in mice is accompanied by the massive accumulation of eosinophils and macrophages (Lammas et al., 1990). Their impaired capacity to present antigens (Jenkins et al., 1990), and inability to restrict infection rate, indicate that they became alternatively activated (unpublished observations). We have shown previously that non-specific effector functions of macrophages - phagocytosis and respiratory burst are gradually suppressed in the course of infection and that low doses of PZQ (60 mg/kg b.w.) in liposomes led to the significant activation of both functions. In further experiments, where infected mice received a much higher total dose of PZQ (see above) and co-administration of SIL was also evaluated, phagocytic activity of peritoneal macrophages was temporarily suppressed following termination of therapy, more in PZQ-treated group (Table 6). However, production of superoxide anions by adherent peritoneal cells was suppressed only in the group treated with PZQ and SIL gradually reaching values found in non-infected mice (Velebný et al., 2010). The mechanism underlying this effect of drugs on non-specific functions is unknown, and fits to the theory that SIL has anti-inflammatory activity. In the liver with *S. mansoni* induced fibrosis, El-Lakkany et al. (2012) found significant reduction of mast cell numbers and tissue expression of TGF-β1 following SIL administration. Immunomodulatory activity of silymarin on T cell responses was demonstrated in many studies with controversial findings, so it is likely that polarisation of Th1 versus Th2 immune balance following silymarin treatment is disease-specific. For example, in case of OVA-antigen sensitized mice, treatment enhanced production of Th1 type cytokine IFN-γ and decreased production of IL-4, which may be a beneficial effect against IgE-mediated allergy (Kuo and Jan, 2009). On the other hand, in Con-A induced hepatitis in mice, silibinin suppressed expression of TNF-α, IFN-γ, IL-12 and IL-4, whereas IL-10 synthesis was augmented (Schumann et al., 2003). In our experiment on the mouse - *M. vogae* model, in peritoneal cavity co-administration of SIL with PZQ enhanced the larvicidal effect of drug

(Hrčkova and Velebný, 2012) and markedly modulated proportions of all inflammatory cell types in comparison with controls.

Table 6. Phagocytic activity of peritoneal macrophages obtained during follow-up therapy from *Mesocestoides vogae* infected mice after oral administration of praziquantel (PZQ) alone or in combination with silymarin (SIL)

Days p.i/ p.t	Experimental groups of mice		
	Control	PZQ	PZQ+SIL
25/ 1	63.2 ± 3.0	39.4 ± 2.0*	52.3 ± 1.7*
28/ 4	61.0 ± 3.1	47.5 ± 1.8*	65.3 ± 2.6
35/ 11	59.3 ± 2.8	62.1 ± 3.4	63.5 ± 1.2§
44/ 20	55.4 ± 2.4	63.4 ± 1.3	64.1 ± 3.2§

Legend: * Significantly lower value in comparison with control-untreated group, ($P < 0.05$). Data are expressed as mean ± SD, (n=4).

§ Significantly higher value in comparison with control-untreated group, ($P < 0.05$).

PZQ was given in 10 daily doses (total dose was 350 mg/kg b.w.) between days 15-24.

Silymarin was given in 10 daily doses (total dose was 300 mg/kg b.w.) between days 15-24 p.i.

Phagocytic activity was calculated as proportion (%) of cells containing three and more HEMA particles from each 100 counted cells, in total 400 cells were counted for each group.

We conclude that in the chronic liver diseases caused by helminth infections, combined therapy with the antihelmintic drug PZQ and the flavonoid antioxidant silymarin, could be a future alternative treatment. The main beneficial effect of silymarin-co-administration is the potentiation of the larvicidal action of the drug, which is mediated indirectly via its antioxidant capacity, modulating the chronic inflammatory reactions that results in the down-regulation of fibrogenesis and thus higher availability of antihelmintic drug for parasites. Regarding the synergistic effect of SIL with praziquantel in therapy of larval cestodoses, immunomodulatory activity of this remarkable flavonoid has to be also considered and awaits further study.

Acknowledgments

We would like to express our deep gratitude to Prof. Chris Arme (Keele University, United Kingdom) for his help in the manuscript preparation.

The main support for this work was provided by the Scientific Grant Agency VEGA of the Ministry of Education and the Slovak Academy of Sciences (Project no. 2/0150/13). The technical support for the realization of this work was provided within the frame of the project 'Centrum of Excellence for Parasitology' No. 26220120022 supported by the operating programme 'Research and Development' funded by the European Fund for Regional Development (0.3).

References

Abraham, K.M. and Teale, J.M. (1987). Isotype restriction during infection of mice with the cestode *Mesocestoides corti*: role of immune suppression. *Journal of Immunology, 138,* 1699-1704.

Akbarieh, M., Tawashi, R., Ghorab, M., and Kassem, M. (1991). Praziquantel as prophylactic in Schistosomiasis: Formulation and stability evaluation of a liposomal delivery system. *Temporal Control of Drug Delivery. Annals of the New York Academy of Sciences*, *618*, 572-574.

Allen, T.M. and Cullis, P.R. (2013). Liposomal drug delivery systems: From concept to clinical applications. *Advanced Drug Delivery Reviews 65,* 36–48.

Anthony, R.M, Rutitzky L.I., Urban, J.F., Stadecker, M.J. and Gause, W.C. (2007). Protective immune mechanisms in helminth infections. *Nature Reviews Immunology*, *7*, 975-987.

Aragon, A.D., Imani, R.A., Blackburn, V.R., Cupit, P.M., Melman, S.D., Goronga, T., Webb, T., Loker, E.S. and Cunningham C. (2009). Towards understanding of the mechanism of action of praziquantel. *Molecular and Biochemical Parasitology, 164*, 57-65.

Bagrade, D., Šnábel, V., Romig, T., Ozolinš, J., Hüttner, M., Miterpáková, M., Ševcová, D. and Dubinský, P. (2008). *Echinococcus multilocularis* is a frequent parasite of red foxes (*Vulpes vulpes*) in Latvia. *Helminthologia, 45,* 157-161.

Baird, R.A., Wiebe, S., Zunt, J.R., Halperin, J.J., Gronseth, G. and Roos K.L. (2013). Evidence-based guideline: Treatment of paranchymal neurocysticercosis. *Neurology, 80,* 1424-1429.

Baroni, G.S., D´Ambrosio, L., Farretti, G., Casini, A., Di Sario, A., Salzano, R., Ridolfi, F., Saccomanno, S., Jezequel, A.M. and Benedetti, A. (1998). Fibrogenic effect of oxidative stress on rat hepatic stellate cells. *Hepatology, 27*, 720-726.

Brossard, M., Andreutti, C. and Siegenthaler, M. (2007). Infection of red foxes with *Echinococcus multiloccularis* in western Switzerland. *Journal of Helmintholopgy, 81*: 369-376.

Bygott, J.M. and Chiodini, P.L. (2009). Praziquantel: Neglected drug? Ineffective treatment? Or therapeutic choice in cystic hydatid disease? *Acta Tropica, 111*, 95–101.

Cardona, A.E., Restrepo, B.I., Jaramillo, J.M. and Teale J.M. (1999). Development of an animal model for neurocysticercosis: immune response in the central nervous system is characterized by a predominance of T-cells. *Journal of Immunology*, 162, 995-1002.

Choi, W.Y., Kim, B.C. and Choi, H.S. (1967). The first case of human infection with tapeworms of the genus *Mesocestoides* in Korea. *Korean Journal of Parasitology, 5,* 21-23.

Chen, Y., Dong, L., Weng, D., Liu, F., Song, L., Li, C., Tang, W. and Chen, J. (2013). 1,3-β-glucan affects the balance of Th1/Th2 cytokines by promoting secretion of anti-imflammatory cytokines in vitro. *Molecular Medicine Reports, 2013-06-25. http://scholar.qsensei.com/content/1w2kkc /index#details*

Chu, D., Luo, Q., Li, C., Gao, Z., Yu, L., Wei, W., Wu, Q. and Shen, J. (2007). Paeoniflorin inhibits TGF-β1-mediated collagen production by *Schistosoma japonicum* soluble egg antigen in vitro. *Parasitology, 134*, 1611-1621.

Chu, D., Du, M., Hu, X., Wu, Q. and Shen, J. (2011). Paeoniflorin attenuates schistosomiasis japonica-associated liver fibrosis through inhibition alternative activation of macrophages. *Parasitology, 138,* 1259-1271.

Cioli, D. and Pica-Mattocia, L. (2003). Praziquantel. *Parasitology Research, 90,* S3-9.

Coyle, C.M, Mahanty, S., Zunt, J.R., Wallin, M.T., Cantey, P.T., White, A.C. Jr., O ´Neal, S.E., Serpa, J.A., Southern, P.M., Wilkins, P., McCarthy, A.E., Higgs, E.S. and Nash, T.E. (2012). Neurocysicercosis: neglected but not forgotten. *PloS Neglected Tropical Diseases, 6*: e1500.

Craig, P. (2003). *Echinococcus multilocularis. Current Opinion in Infectious Diseases, 16,* 437-444.

Crommelin, D.J.A., Eling, W.M.C., Steerenberg, P.A., Nassander, U.K., Storm, G., De Jong, W.H., Van Hoese, Q.G.C.M. and Zuidema, J. (1991). Liposomes and immunoliposomes for controlled release or site specific delivery of anti-parasitic drugs and cytostatics. *Journal of Controlled Release,* 16, 147- 154.

Crosbie, P.R., Boyce, W.M., Platzer, E.G., Nadler, S.A. and Kerner, C. (1998). Diagnostic procedures and treatment of eleven dogs with peritoneal infections caused by *Mesocestoides* spp. *Journal of the American Vetrinary Medicine Association, 213,* 1578-1583.

Dachman, W.D., Adubofour, K.O., Bikin, D.S., Johnson, C.H., Mullin, P.D. and Winograd, M. (1994). Cimetidine-induced rise in praziquantel levels in a patient with neurocysticercosis being treated with anticonvulsants. *Journal of Infectious Diseases, 169*, 689–691.

Date, A.A., Joshi, M.D. and Patravale, V.B. (2007). Parasitic diseases: Liposomes and polymeric nanoparticles versus lipid nanoparticles. *Advanced Drug Delivery Reviews,* 59, 505–521.

Dautović-Krkić, S., Huskić, J., Cengić, D., Dizdarević, S. et al. (2002). Praziquantel in the prevention of recurrence of human echinococcosis. *Medicinski Arhiv, 56*, 263-266 (in Croatian).

Dayan, A.D. (2003). Albendazole, mebendazole and praziquantel. Review of non-clinical toxicity and pharmacokinetics. *Acta Tropica*, *86*, 141-159

De Blesser, P.J., Xu, G., Romboust, K., Rogiers, V. and Geerts, A. (1999). Glutathione levels discriminate between oxidative stress and transforming growth factor-β signalling in activated rat hepatic stellate cells. *Journal of Biological Chemistry, 274,* 33881-33887.

Ditteová, G., Velebný, S. and Hrčková, G. (2003). Modulation of liver fibrosis and pathophysiologic changes in mice infected with *Mesocestoides corti* (*M. vogae*) after administration of glucan and liposomized glucan in combination with vitamin C. *Journal of Helminthology*, *77*, 219-226.

Ditteová, G., Velebný, S. and Hrčková, G. (2005). The dose dependent effect of glucan on worm burden and pathology of mice infected with *Mesocestoides corti (M.vogae)* tetrathyridia. *Helminthologia, 40*, 123-130.

Dvorožňáková, E., Porubcová, J., Šnábel, V. and Fedoročko, P. (2008). Immunomodulative effect of liposomized muramyltripeptide phosphatidylethanolamine (L-MTP-PE) on mice with alveolar echinococcosis and treated with albendazole. *Parasitology Research, 103,* 919-929.

Dvorožňáková, E., Porubcová, J. and Ševčíková, Z. (2009). Immune response of mice with alveolar echinococcosis to therapy with transfer factor, alone and in combination with albendazole. *Parasitology Research, 105,* 1067-1076.

Eckert, J., Schantz, P.M., Gasser, R.B., Torgerson, P.R., Bessonov, A.S., Movsessian, S.O., Thakur, A., Grimm, F. and Nikogosian, M.A. (2001a). Geographic distribution and prevalence. In: J. Eckert, M.A. Gemmel, F.X.

Messlin and Z.S. Pawlowski (Eds.), *WHO/OIE Manual on echinococcosis in humans and animals: a public helth problem of global concern.*(pp. 101-143, Chapter 4). Paris, France: World Organisation for Animal Health.

Eckert, J., Deplazes, P., Craig, P.S., Gemmel, M.A., Gottstein, B., Heath, D., Jenkins, D.J., Kamiya, M. and Lightowlers, M. (2001b). Echinococcus in animals: clinical aspects, diagnosis and treatment. In: J. Eckert, M.A. Gemmel, F.X. Messlin and Z.S. Pawlowski (Eds.), *WHO/OIE Manual on echinococcosis in humans and animals: a public helth problem of global concern.*(pp. 73-100, Chapter 3). Paris, France: World Organisation for Animal Health.

El-Lakkany, N.M., Hammam, O.A., El-Maadawy, W.H., Badawy, A.A., Ain-Shoka, A.A. and Ebeid, F.A. (2012). Anti-inflammatory/anti-fibrotic effects of the hepatoprotective silymarin and the schistosomicide praziquantel against *Schistosoma mansoni*-induced liver fibrosis. *Parasites & Vectors, 5*, art.no.9.

Eleni, C., Scaramozzino, P., Busi, M., Ingrosso, S., D´Amelio, S. and De Liberato, C. (2007). Proliferative peritoneal and pleural cestodiasis in a cat caused by metacestodes of *Mesocestoides* sp. Anatomohistopathological findings and genetic identification. *Parasite, 14,* 71-76.

EMEA-European Medicines Evaluation Agency (1996).Praziquantel Summary Report by CVMP. EMEA/MRL/141/96 September 1996. *EMEA, London.*

EMEA-European Medicines Evaluation Agency (1997). Albendazole Summary Report by CVMP. EMEA/MRL/247/97-Final. *EMEA, London.*

EMEA-European Medicines Evaluation Agency (1999). Mebendazole Summary. Report by CVMP. EMEA/MRL/625/99-Final. July 1999. *EMEA, London.*

EMEA-European Medicines Evaluation Agency (2001). Mebendazole Summary Report 2 by CVMP. EMEA/MRL/781/01-Final. March 2001. *EMEA, London.*

Eom, K.S., Kim, S.H.and Rim, H.J. (1988). Efficacy of praziquantel (Cesocide injection) in treatment of cestode infections in domestic and laboratory animals. *Korean Journal of Parasitology, 26*, 121-126,

Escobar, A. (1983). The pathology of neurocysticercosis. In: E. Palacios, J. Rodriguez-Carbajal and J.M. Taveras (Eds.), *Cysticercosis of the Central Nervous System* (pp. 27-54). Springfield, IL: Charles C. Thomas.

Etges, F.J. (1991). The proliferative tetrathyridium of *Mesocesoides vogae* sp. n. (Cestoda). *Journal of the Helminthological Society of Wasington, 58*, 181-185.

European Comission (2000).Opinion of the scientific comittee on veterinary measures relating to public health on the control of taeniosis/cysticercosis in man and animals. http://ec.europa.eu/food/fs/sc/scv/out36_en.pdf

Fallon, P.G., Sturrock, R.F., Niang, A.C. and Doenhoff, M.J. (1995). Short report: diminished susceptibility to praziquantel in a Senegal isolate of *Schistosoma mansoni. American Journal of Tropical Medicine and Hygiene, 53*, 61-62.

Fan, S.Q. (1988). First case of *Mesocestoides lineatus* infection in China (in Chinese). *Chinese Journal of Parasitology and Parasitic Diseases. 64,* 310.

Friedman, S.L. (2000). Molecular regulation of hepatic fibrosis, an integrated cellular response to tissue injury. *Journal of Biological Chemistry, 275*, 2247-2250.

Fuentes, M.V., Galàn-Puchades, M.T. and Malone, J. (2003). A new case report of human *Mesocestoides* infection in the United States. *American Journal of Tropical Medicine and Hygiene, 68,* 566-567.

Garcia, H.H, Evans, C.A., Nash, T.E., Takayanagui, O.M., White, A.C. Jr., et al. (2002). Current consensus guidelines for treatment of neurocysticercosis. *Clinical Microbiology Rev*iews, *15*, 747-756.

Garcia, H.H., Gonzales, A.E. and Gilman, R.H. (2011). Cysticercosis of the central nervous system – how should it be managed. *Current Opinion in Infectious Diseases, 24,* 423-427.

Geary, T.G., Woo, K., McCarthy, J.S., Mackenzie, C.D., Horton, J. et al. (2010). Unresolved issues in anthelmintic pharmacology for helminthiases in humans. *International Journal for Parasitology, 40,* 1-13.

Gharagozloo, M., Velardi, E., Bruscoli, S., Agostini, M., Di Sante, M., Donato, V. Amirghofran, Z. and Riccardi, C. (2010). Silymarin suppress $CD4^{+}T$ cell activation and proliferation: Effects on NFκB activity and IL-2 production. *Pharmacological Research, 61,* 405-409.

Goyal, P., Goyal, K., Kumar, S.G., Singh, A., Katare, O.P. and Mishira, D.N. (2005). Liposomal drug delivery systems – Clinical applications. *Acta Pharmacologica, 55*, 1-25.

Gregoriadis, G. (1977). Targeting of drug. *Nature, 265*, 407-411.

Guerret, S., Vuitton, D.A., Liance, M. and Pater, C. (1998). *Echinococcus multilocularis*: relationship between susceptibility/resistance and liver fibrogenesis in experimental mice. *Parasitology Research, 84*, 657-667.

Havsteen, B.H. (2002). The biochemistry and medical significance of the flavonoids. *Pharmacology & Therapeutics, 96,* 67-202.

Herre, J., Gordon, S. and Brown, G.D. (2004). Dectin-1 and its role in the recognition of β-glucans by macrophages. *Molecular Immunology, 40,* 869-876.

Hirano, K. and Hunt, C.A. (1985). Lymphatic transport of liposome-encapsulated agents: effects of liposome size following intraperitoneal administration. *Journal of Pharmaceutical Sciences, 74,* 915-921.

Homeida, M., Leahy, W., Copeland, S., Ali, M.M. and Harron, D.W. (1994). Pharmacokinetic interaction between praziquantel and albendazole in Sudanese men. *Annals of Tropical Medicine and Parasitology, 88,* 551–559.

Horton, R.J. (1997). Albendazole in the treatment of human cystic echinococcosis. *Acta Tropica, 64*, 79–93.

Hrčkova, G. and Velebný, S. (1995). Effects of free and liposomized praziquantel on worm burden and antibody response in mice infected with *Mesocestoides corti* tetrathyridia. *Journal of Helminthology, 69,* 213-221.

Hrčkova, G. and Velebný, S. (1997). Effect of praziquantel and liposome-incorporated praziquantel on peritoneal macrophage activation in mice infected with *Mesocestoides corti* tetrathyridia (Cestoda). *Parasitology, 114*, 475-482.

Hrčkova, G., Velebný, S. and Dezfuli, B.S. (1998). Entrapment of praziquantel in liposomes modifies effects of drug on morphology and motility of *Mesocestoides corti* (syn. *vogae*) tetrathyridia (Cestoda) in mice. *Helminthologia*, *35*, 13-20.

Hrčkova, G., Velebný, S. and Giboda, M. (2000). Distribution of [^{3}H]cholesterol-labelled liposomes with or without praziquantel in mice infected with *Mesocestoides corti* (Cestoda) tetrathyridia. *Comparative Biochemistry and Physiology Part C, 126,* 167-174.

Hrčkova, G., Velebný, S., Daxnerová, Z. and Solár, P. (2006). Praziquantel and liposomized-glucan treatment modulated liver fibrogenesis and mastocytosis in mice infected with *Mesocestoides vogae* (*M.corti*, Cestoda) tetrathyridia. *Parasitology*, *132*, 581-594.

Hrčkova, G., Velebný, S. and Solár, P. (2010). Dynamics of hepatic stellate cells, collagen types I and III synthesis and gene expression of selected cytokines during hepatic fibrogenesis following *Mesocestoides vogae* (Cestoda) infection in mice. *International Journal for Parasitology*, *40,* 163-174.

Hrčkova, G., Miterpáková, M., O´Connor, A., Šnábel, V. and Olson, P.D. (2011). Molecular and morphological circumscription of *Mesocestoides* tapeworms from red foxes (*Vulpes vulpes*) in central Europe. *Parasitology, 138*, 638-647.

Hrčkova, G. and Velebný, S. (2012). Current situation and new possibilities in pharmacology of parasitic infections. In *Recent researches in medicine & medical chemistry: Proceedings. Kos Island, Greece, July 14-17, 2012.* Carlos Rivas-Echeveria, Corina Carranca (Eds.). Kos : WSEAS Press, 2012, p. 106-112. ISBN 978-1-61804-111-1. ISSN 1790-5125.

Hrčkova, G. and Velebný, S. (2013). Pharmacological potential of selected natural compounds in the control of parasitic diseases. Wien, Heidelberg, New York, Dordrecht and London: Springer. ISBN 978-3-7091-1324-0.

Irizarry-Rovira, A.R., Wolf, A. and Bolek, M. (2007). *Taenia taeniaeformis*-induced metastatic hepatic sarcoma in a pet rat (*Rattus norvegicus*) *Journal of Exotic Pet Medicine, 16,* 45-48.

Jenkins, P., Dixon, J.B., Rakha, N.K. and Carter, S.D. (1990). Regulation of macrophage-medited larvicidal activity in *Echinococcus granulosus* and *Mesocestoides corti* (Cestoda) infection in mice. *Parasitology,* 100, 309-315.

Jenkins, P., Dixon, J.B., Haywood, S., Rakha, N.K. and Carter, S.D. (1991). Differential regulation of murine *Mesocestoides corti* infection by bacterial lipopolysaccharide and intrferon-γ. *Parasitology, 102*, 125-132.

Jiménez-Mejías, M.E., Alarcón-Cruz, J.C., Márquez-Rivas, F.J. et al. (2000). Orbital hydatid cyst: treatment and prevention of recurrences with albendazole plus praziquantel. *Journal of Infection, 41,* 105-107.

Jung, H., Medina, R., Castro, N., Corona, T. and Sotelo, J. (1997). Pharmacokinetic study of praziquantel administered alone and in combination with cimetidine in a single-day therapeutic regimen. *Antimicrobial Agents and Chemotherapy, 41,* 1526-1529.

Kogan, G., Alföldi, J. and Masler, L. (1988). Carbon-13 NMR spectroscopic investigation of two yeast cell wall β-D-glucans. *Biopolymers, 27*, 1055-1063.

Kohn, A.B., Roberts-Misterly, J.M., Anderson, P.A.V. and Greenberg, R.M. (2003). Creation by mutagenesis of a mammalian Ca^{2+} channel β subunit that confers praziquantel sensitivity to a mammalian Ca^{2+} channel. *International Journal for Parasitology., 33*, 1303-1308.

Kraft, R. (2007). Cysticercosis: an emerging parasitic disease. *American Family Physician, 76, 91-96.*

Kuo, F.H. and Jan, T.R. (2009). Silybinin attenuates antigen-specific IgE production through the modulation of Th1/Th2 balance in ovalbumin-sensitized BALB/c mice. *Phytomedicine, 16,* 271-276.

Lammas, D.A., Mitchell, L.A. and Wakelin, D. (1990). Genetic influences upon eosinophilia and resistance in mice infected with *Mesocestoides corti. Parasitology, 101,* 291-299.

Literák, L., Olson, P.D., Georgiev, B.B. and Špakulová, M. (2004). First record of metacestodes of *Mesocestoides* sp. in the common starling (*Sturmus vulgaris*) in Europe, with an 18S rDNA characterization of the isolate. *Folia Parasitologica, 51*, 45-49.

Liu, Y.H. (1984). *Natl. Med. J. China, 64,*243-247. Cited in Sui, F., Xiao, S.and Catto, X. (1988). Clinical use of praziquantel in China. *Parasitology Today, 4,* 312-315.

Lv, H.L., Peng, X.Y., Zhang, S.J., Aduwayi, Yang, H.Q., Sun, H., Yang, J., Li, B.J. and Liu, Y.K. (2008). Effect of the liposome albendazole and Huai-Er fungus extract on hepatic infection of *Echinococcus granulosus* in mice. *Zhongguo Ji Sheng Chong Xue Yu Ji Sheng Chong Bing Za Zhi, 26,* 361-365.

Maizels, R.M., Balic, A., Gomez-Escobar, N., Nair, M., Taylor, M.D. and Allen J.E. (2004). Helminth parasites – masters of regulation. *Immunological Rev*iews, *201*, 89-116.

Majtán, J., Kogan, G., Kováčová, E. Bíliková, K. and Šimúth J. (2005). Stimulation of TNF-α release by fungal cell wall polysaccharides. *Zeitschrift für Naturforshung, 60c*, 921-926.

Manfredi, M.T., Di Cerbo, A.R., Zanzani, S., Moriggia, A., Fattori, D., Siboni, A., Bonazza, V., Filice, C. and Brunetti, E. (2011). Prevalence of echinococcosis in humans, livestock and dogs in northern Italy. *Helminthologia, 48,* 59-66.

Marchiondo, A. A., Ming, R., Andersen, F. L., Slusser, J. H. and Conder, G. A. (1994). Enhanced larval cyst growth of *E. multitilocalaris* in praziquantel-treated jids. *American Journal of Tropical Medicine and Hygiene, 50,* 120-127.

Matthaiou, D.K., Panos, G., Adamidi, E.S. and Falagas, M.E. (2008). Albendazole versus Praziquantel in the Treatment of Neurocysticercosis: A Meta-analysis of Comparative Trials. *PLoS Neglected Tropical Diseases*, *2*, e194.

McAllister, C.T., Bruce Conn, D., Feed, P.S. and Burdick, D.A. (1991). A new host and locality record for *Mesocestoides* sp. tetrathyridia (Cestoidea: Cyclophyllidea), with a summary of the genus from snakes of the wold. *Journal of Parasitology, 77,* 329-331.

McManus, D.P., Gray, D.J., Zhang, W. and Yang, Y. (2012). Diagnosis, treatment and management of echinococcosis. *British Medical Journal, 344,* e3866.

Mehlhorn, B., Becker, B., Andrews, P., Thomas, H. and Frenkel, J.K. (1981). In vivo and in vitro experiments on the effects of praziquantel on *Schistosoma mansoni*. A light and electron microscopic study. *Arzneilmittelforschung, 31*, 544-554.

Middleton, E., Kandaswami, C.H. and Theoharides, T.C. (2000). The effects of plant flavonoids on mammalian cells: Implications for inflammation, heart disease, and cancer. *Pharmacology Reviews, 52*, 673-751.

Mitchell, G.F., Marchalonis, J.J., Smith, P.M., Nicholas, W.L. and Warner, N.L. (1977). Studies on immune response to larval cestodes in mice. Immunoglobulins associated with the larvae of *Mesocestoides corti. Australian Journal of Experimental Biology and Medical Science, 55,* 187-211.

Miterpaková, M. and Dubinský, P. (2011). Fox tapeworm (*Echinococcus multilocularis*) in Slovakia – summarizing the long-term monitoring. *Helminthologia, 48,* 155-161.

Monroe, J.G., Haldar, S., Prystowsky, M.B. and Lammie, P. (1988). Lymphokine regulation of inflammatory processes: interleukin-4 stimulates fibroblast proliferation. *Clinical Immunology and Immunopathology, 49,* 292-298.

Montero, R. and Ostrosky, P. (1997). Genotoxic activity of praziquantel. *Mutation Research, 387*, 123-139.

Moreno, M.J., Urrea-Paris, M.A., Casado, N. and Rodriguez-Caabeiro, F. (2001). Praziquantel and albendazole in the combined treatment of experimental hydatid disease. *Parasitology Research, 87,* 235-238.

Morris, D.L., Richards, K.S. and Chinnery, J.B. (1986). Protoscolicidal effect of praziquantel – in vitro and electron microscopical studies on *Echinococcus granulosus. Journal of Antimicrobial Chemotherapy, 18,* 687-691.

Morris, D.L., Chinnery, J.B., Georgiou, G., Stamatakis, G. and Golematis, B. (1987). Penetration of albendazole sulphoxide into hydatid cysts. *Gut, 28,* 75–80.

Morris, D.L., Taylor, D., Daniels, E.M., Riley, E. and Richards, K.S. (1988). Determination of the minimum length of praziquantel therapy required for the in vitro treatment of protoscoleces of *Echinococcus granulosus. Journal of Helminthology, 62,* 10-14.

Morris, D.L., Richards, K.S., Cklarkson, M.J. and Taylor, D. (1990). Comparison of albendazole and praziquantel therapy of *Echinococcus granulosus* in naturally infected sheep. *Veterinary Parasitology, 36,* 83-90.

Morista, T., Nagase, K., Moriyama, K. and Matumoto, Z. (1975). The 11th case of human infection with *Mesocestoides lineatus* in Japan. *Japanesse Journal of Parasitology, 24,* 353-356.

Mourão, S.C., Costa, P.I., Salgado, H.R.N. and Gremiao, M.P.D. (2005). Improvement of antischistosomal activity of praziquantel by incorporation into phosphatidylcholine-containing liposomes. *International Journal of Pharmaceutics, 295*, 157-162.

Municio, C., Alvarez, Y., Montero, O., Hugo, E., Rodriguez, M., Domingo, E., Alonso, S., Fernández, N. and Crespo, M.S. (2013). The response of human macrophages to β-glucans depends on the inflammatory milieu. *PLoS ONE, 8(4),* e2016.

Na-Bangchang, K, Vanijanonta, S. and Karbwang, J. (1995). Plasma concentrations of praziquantel during the therapy of neurocysticecosis with praziquantel, in the presence of antiepileptics and dexamethasone. *Southeast Asian Journal of Tropical Medicine and Public Health, 26*,120-123.

Nagase, K., Kani, A., Totani, T., Hamamoto, T. and Torikai, K. (1983). Report of human case of *Mesocestoides lineatus* and preliminary investigation into infective sources. *Japanese Journal of Parasitology, 32 (Suppl),* 18.

Nichol S., Ball S. J and Snow, K. R. (1981). Prevalence of intestinal parasites in feral cats in some urban areas of England. *Veterinary Parasito*logy, *9,* 107-110.

Niu, R.L., Xue, H.X. and Mo, H.M. (2001). Efficacy of albendazole immunoliposomes against *Echinococcus granulosus* in mice. *Zhongguo Ji Sheng Chong Xue Yu Ji Sheng Chong Bing Za Zhi, 19,* 141-144.

Olds, G.R. (2003). Administration of praziquantel to pregnant and lactating women. *Acta Tropica, 86,* 185-195

Olson, P.D., Yoder, K., Fajardo, L-G L.F., Marty, A.M., van de Pas, S., Olivier, C. and Relman, D.A. (2003). Lethal invasive cestodiasis in immunosuppressed patients. *Journal of Infective Diseases, 187,* 1962-1966.

Olson, P.D. (2008). Hox genes and parasitic flatworms: New opportunities, challenges and lessons from the free living. *Parasitology International, 57,* 8-17.

Palomares, F., Palencia, G., Pérez, R., Gonzáles-Esquivel, D., Castro, N. and Cook, H.J. (2004). In vitro effects of albendazole sulfoxide and praziquantel against *Taenia solium* and *Taenia crassiceps* cysts. *Antimicrobial Agents and Chemotherapy, 48,* 2302-2304.

Palomares, F., Palencia, G., Ambrosio, J.R., Ortiz, A.S. and Jung-Cook, H. (2006). Evaluation of the efficacy of albendazole supphoxide and praziquantel in combination on *Taenia crassiceps* cysts: in vitro studies. *Journal of Antimicrobial Chemotherapy, 57,* 482-488.

Panwar, P., Pandey, B. and Lakhera, P.C. (2010). Preparation, characterization, and in vitro release study of albendazole-encapsulated nanosize liposomes. *International Journal of Nanomedicine, 5,* 101-108.

Papini, R., Matteini, A., Bandinelli, P., Pampurini, F. and Mancianti, F. (2010). Effectiveness of praziquantel for the treatment of peritoneal larval cestodiasis in dogs: A case report. *Veterinary Parasitology, 170*, 158-161.

Piens, M.A., Persat, F., May, F. and Mojon, M. (1989). Praziquantel dans l'hydatidose humaine. *Bulletin de la Socite de Pathologie Exotique et de ses Filiales, 82*, 503-512.

Porubcová, J., Dvorožňáková, E. and Ševčíková, Z. (2007). Immunomodulative effect of glucan and/or glucan supplemented with zinc in albendazole therapy for murine alveolar echinococcosis. *Parasitology Research, 101*, 751-760.

Prichard, R.K., Basáñez , M.G., Boatin, B.A., McCarthy, J.S., García, H.H. et al. (2012). A research agenda for helminth diseases of humans: intervention for control and elimination. *PLoS Neglected Tropical Diseases, 6,* e1549

Puxeddu, I., Piliponsky, A.M., Bachelet, I. and Levi-Schaffer, F. (2003). Cells in focus. Mast cells in allergy and beyond. *International Journal of Biochemistry and Cell Biology, 35,* 1601-1607.

Rajshekhar, V., Joshi, D.D., Doanh, N.Q., van De, N. and Xiaonong, Z. (2003). *Taenia solium* taeniosis/cysticercosis in Asia: epidemiology, impact and issues. *Acta Tropica, 87,* 53-60.

Rausch, R.L. (1994). Family *Mesocestoididae* Fuhrmann, 1907. In: L.F. Khalil, A. Jones and R.A. Bray (Eds.), *Keys to the cestode parasites of vertebrates* (pp. 309-314). Wallingford, Oxon, UK: CAB International.

Reuter, S. Jensen, B., Buttenschoen, K., Kratzer, W. and Kern, P. (2000). Benzimidazoles in the treatment of alveolar echinococcosis: a comparative study and a review of literature. *Journal of Antimicrobial Chemotherapy, 46,* 451-456.

Reves, H.L. and Friedman, S.L. (2002). Activation of hepatic stelate cells – a key issue in liver fibrosis. *Frontiers in Bioscience, 7,* D808-D826.

Reyes, J.L. and Terrazas, L.I. (2007). The divergent roles of alternatively activated macrophages in helminthic infections. *Parasite Immunology, 29*, 609-619.

Rice, P.J., Kelley, J.L., Kogan, G., Ensley, H.E., Kalbfeisch, J.H., Browder, W.I. and Williams, D.L. (2002). Human monocyte scavenger receptors are pattern recognition receptors for (1-3)-β-D-glucans. *Journal of Leucocyte Biology, 72*, 140-146.

Riganò, R., Buttari, B., De Falco, E., Profumo, E., Ortona, E., Margutti, P., Scottà, C., Teggi, A. and Siracusano, A. (2004). *Echinococcus granulosus*-specific T-cell lines derived from patients at various clinical stages of cystic echinococcosis. *Parasite Immunology, 26,* 45-52.

Roberts, M.G. and Aubert, M.F.A. (1995). A model for the control of *Echinococcus multilocularis* in France. *Vetrinary Parasitology, 56*, 67-74.

Ruenwongsa, P. and Thamavit, W. (1983). Increased efficacy of liposome-encapsulated praziquantel in treatment of opistorchiasis in hamsters. *The Southeast Asian Journal of Tropical Medicine and Publuic Health, 14,* 501-504.

Santos-Magalhaes, N.S., Mosqueira, V.C. (2010). Nanotechnology applied to the treatment of malaria. *Advances Drug Delivery Review, 62*, 560-575.

Schepers, H., Brasseur, R., Goormaghtigh, E., Duquenoy, P. and Ruysschaert, J.M. (1988). Mode of insertion of praziquantel and derivatives into lipid membranes. *Biochemical Pharmacology, 37,* 1615-1623.

Schelling, U., Frank, W., Will, R., Romig, T. and Lucius, R. (1997). Chemotherapy with praziquantel has the potential to reduce the prevalence of *Echinococcus multilocularis* in wild foxes (*Vulpes vulpes*). *Annals of Tropical Medicine and Parasitology, 91*, 179-186.

Shao, Y., Liu, W. and Wen, H. (1999). Effect of liposomal albendazole on the utrastructure of *Echinococcus granulosus* cysts in mice. *Zhongguo Ji Sheng Chong Xue Yu Ji Sheng Chong Bing Za Zhi, 17,* 292-293.

Šoltýs, J., Borošková, Z., Dubinský, P., Tomašovičová, O., Auer, H. and Aspöck, H. (1996). Effect of glucan immunomodulator on the immune response and larval burdens in mice with experimental toxocariosis. *Applied Parasitology, 37*, 161-167.

Sotelo, J. and Del Bruto, O. (2002). Review of neurocysticercosis. *Neurosurgical Focus, 12,* 1-7.

Specht, D. and Vogae, M. (1965). Asexual multiplication of *Mesocestoides* tetrathyridia in laboratory animals. *Journal of Parasitology, 51*, 268-272.

Spicher, M., Naguleswaran, A., Ortega-Mora, L., Müller, J., Gottstein, B. et al. (2008). In vitro and in vivo effects of 2-methoxyestradiol, either alone or combined with albendazole, against *Echinococcus* metacestodes. *Experimental Parasitology, 119,* 475-482.

Steiner, K., Garbe, A., Dickmann, H.W. and Nowak, H. (1976). The fate of praziquantel in the organism. I. Pharmacokinetics in animals. *European Journal of Drug Metabolism and Pharmacokinetics, 2,* 85-95.

Schümann, J., Prockl J., Kiemer, A.K. et al. (2003). Silybinin protects mice from T cell dependent liver injury. *Journal of Hepatology, 39*, 333-340.

Taylor, D., Morris, D. and Richards, K. (1988). Combination chemotherapy of *Echinococcus granulosus* – in vitro studies. *Transactions of the Royal Society of Tropical Medicine and Hygiene, 82,* 263-264.

Taylor, D. and Morris, D. (1988). In vitro culture *of Echinococcus multilocularis* protoscolicidal action of praziquantel and albendazole sulphoxide. *Transactions of the Royal Society of Tropical Medicine and Hygiene, 82,* 265-267.

Taylor, P.R., Brown, G.D., Reid, D.M., Willment, J.A. Martinez-Pomares, L., Gordon, S. and Wong, S,Y.C. (2002). The β-glucan receptor, dectin-1, is predominantly expressed on the surface of cells of the monocyte/macrophage and neutrophil lineages. Journal *of Immunology, 169,* 3876-3882.

Thomas, H., Andrews, P. and Mehlhorn, H. (1982). New results on the effect of praziquantel in experimental cysticercosis. *American Journal of Tropical Medicine and Hygiene, 31*, 803-810.

Thomas, H. and Gönnert, R. (1977). The efficacy of praziquantel against cestodes in animals. *Zeitschrift für Parasitenkunden, 52*, 117-127.

Todd, K.S. Jr., Simond, J. and Dipietro, J.A. (1978). Pathological changes in mice infected with tetrathyridia of *Mesocestoides corti. Laboratory Animals, 12,* 51-53.

Toplu, N., Yildiz, K. and Tunay, R. (2004). Massive cystic tetrathyridiosis in a dog. *Journal of Small Animal Practice, 45,* 410-412.

Torgerson, P.R., Keller, K., Magnotta, M. and Ragland, N. (2010). The global burden of alveolar echinococcosis. *PLoS Neglected Tropical Diseases, 4(6),* e722.

Tsiapali, E., Whaley, S., Kalbfleisch, J., Ensley, H.E., Browder, I.W. and Williams, D.L. (2001). Glucan exhibit weak antioxidant activity, but stimulate macrophage free radical activity. *Free Radical Biology and Medicine, 30*, 393-402.

Urrea-Paris, M.A., Moreno, M.J., Casado, N. and Rodrıguez-Caabeiro, F. (1999). *Echinococcus granulosus*: praziquantel treatment against the metacestode stage. *Parasitology Research 85,* 999– 1006.

Urrea-Paris, M.A., Moreno, M.J., Casado, N. and Rodrıguez-Caabeiro, F. (2000). In vitro effect of praziquantel and albendazole combination therapy in the larval stage of *Echinococcus granulosus. Parasitoogyl Research, 86,* 957–964.

Urrea-Paris, M.A., Moreno, M.J., Casado, N. and Rodriguez-Caabeiro, F. (2002). Relationship between the efficacy of praziquantel treatment and the cystic differentiation in vivo of *Echinococcus granulosus* metacestode. *Parasitology Research, 88*, 26–31.

Várady, M., Konigová, A., Čerňanská, D., Čorba, J. (2005). Effect of combined therapy of an anthelmintic and an immunomodulator on the elimination of gastrointestinal nematodes in sheep. *Helminthologia, 42*, 133-136.

Varin, A. and Gordon, S. (2009). Alternative activation of macrophages: immune function and cellular biology. *Immunobiology, 214*, 630-641.

Velebný, S., Hrčkova, G. and Kogan, G. (2008). Impact of treatment with praziquantel, silymarin and/or β-glucan on pathophysiological markers of liver damage and fibrosis in mice infected with *Mesocestides vogae* (Cestoda) tetrathyridia. *Journal of Helminthology, 82*, 211-219.

Velebný, S., Hrčkova, G., and Königová, A. (2010). Reduction of oxidative stress and liver injury following silymarin and praziquantel treatment in mice with *Mesocestoides vogae* (Cestoda) infection. *Parasitology International*, *59*, 524-531.

Vetvička, V., Thornton, B.P. and Ross, G.D. (1996). Soluble β-glucan polysaccharide binding to the lectin site of neutrophil or natural killer cell complement receptor type 3 (CD11b/CD18) generates a primed state capable of mediating cytotoxicity of iC3b-opsonized target cells. *Journal of Clinical Investigation, 98,* 50-57.

Vuitton, D.A. (2009). Benzimidazoles for the treatment of cystic and alveollar echinococcosis: what is the consensus? *Expert Review of Anti-Infective Therapy, 72,* 145-149.

Vuitton, D.A. (2003). The ambiguous role of immunity in echinoccosis: protection of the host or of the parasite? *Acta Tropica, 85*, 119-132.

Watson, M. (2009). Praziquantel. *Journal of Exotic Pet Medicine, 18,* 229-231.

Wei, D., Zhang., L., Williams, D.L. and Browder, W. (2002). Glucan stimulates human dermal fibroblasts collagen biosynthesis through a nuclear factor-1 dependent mechanism. *Wound Repair and Regeneration, 10*, 161-168.

Wen, H., New, R.R.C., Muhmut, M., Wang, J.H., Wang, Y.H., Zhang, J.H., Shao, Y.M. and Craig, P.S. (1996). Pharmacology and efficacy of liposome-entrapped albendazole in experimental secondary alveolar echinococcosis and effect of co-administration with cimetidine. *Parasitology, 113,* 111-121.

White, T.R., Thompson, R.C.A., Penhale, W.J. and Chihara, G. (1988). The effect of lentinan on the resistance of mice to *Mesocestoides corti. Parasitology Research, 74,* 563-568.

WHO (1996). Guidliness for treatment of cystic and alveolar echinococcosis in humans. *Bulletin of the World Health Organisation, 74*, 231-242.

WHO (2002). Prevention and control of schistosomiasis and soil-transmitted helminthiasis: report of a WHO expert committee. Technical Report Series 912. Geneva: World Health Organization, pp. 1-57.

WHO (2007). Global plan to combat neglected tropical diseases 2008-2015. *http://whqlibdoc.who.int/hq/2007/who_cds_ntd_2007.3_eng.pdf*

Williams, C.A. and Conn, D.B. (1985). Localization and associated histopathology of asexualay proliferative *Mesocestoides corti* tetrathyridia (Cestoda) infecting mouse mammary glands. *International Journal for Parasitology, 15,* 245-248.

Williams, D.L., Ha, T., Li, C., Laffan, J.J., Kalbfleisch, J.H. and Browder, W. (2000). Inhibition of LPS induced NFκB activation by a glucan ligand involves down regulation of IKKβ kinase activity and altered phosphorylation and degradation of IκBα. *Shock, 13*, 446-452.

Wirtherle, N., Wiemann, A., Ottenjann, M., Linzmann, H., van der Grinten, E., Kohn, B., Gruber, A.D. and Clausen, P.H. (2007). First case of canine peritoneal larval cestodosis caused by *Mesocestoides lineatus* in Germany. *Parasitology International, 56,* 317-320.

Wu, J. and Zern, M.A. (2000). Hepatic stellate cells: a target to the treatment of liver fibrosis. *Journal of Gastroenterology, 35*, 665-672.

Yuan, L. and Kaplowitz, N. (2009). Glutathione in liver diseases and hepatotoxicity, *Molecular Aspects of Medicine, 30*, 29-41.

Yun, C-H., Estrada, A., van Kessel, A., Gajadhar, A.A., Redmond, M.J. and Laarveld, B. (1997). (1-3, 1-4) oat glucan enhances resistance to *Eimeria vermiformis* infection in immunosuppressed mice. *International Journal for Parasitology,* 27, 329-337.

Zafar, M.J. (2013). Neurocysticercosis. *Medscape News and Perspectives* (K.L. Roos, Chief Editor). *http://emedicine.medscape.com/article /1168656-overview#a0156*

Zaleśny, G. and Hildebrand, J. (2011). Molecular identification of *Mesocestoides* spp. from intermediate hosts (rodents) in central Europe (Poland). *Parasitology Research, 110*, 1055-1061.

Zheng, D. Wang, Y., Zhang, D., Liu, Z., Duan, C., Jia, L. Wang, F. Liu, Y., Liu, G., Hao, L. and Zhang, Q. (2011). In vitro antitumour activity of silybin nanosuspension in PC-3 cells. *Cancer Letters, 307,* 158-164.

Zhong, X., Zhu, Y., Lu, Q., Zhang, J., Ge, Z. and Zhong, S. (2006). Silymarin causes caspases activation and apoptosis in K562 leukemia cells through inactivation of Akt pathway. *Toxicology, 227,* 211-216.

In: Anthelmintics
Editor: William Quick
ISBN: 978-1-63117-714-9

Chapter 6

Efficacy of Neem and Pawpaw Products against *Oesophagostomum* Spp Infection in Pigs

***John Maina Kagira*[1,*], *Paul Njuki Kanyari*[2], *Samuel Maina Githigia*[2], *Ng'ang'a Chege*[2] and *Ndicho Maingi*[2]**

[1]Jomo Kenyatta University of Agriculture and Technology, Nairobi, Kenya
[2]Department of Veterinary Pathology, Microbiology and Parasitology, Faculty of Veterinary Medicine, University of Nairobi, Nairobi, Kenya

Abstract

Plant based remedies are used by pig farmers in control of nematode parasites, although their efficacies has not been evaluated under *in-vitro* and *in-vivo* experiments. Pawpaw and neem products are commonly used as anthelmintics by farmers in Kenya to control of livestock nematodes. The current study evaluated the efficacy of these products using *in-vitro* and *in-vivo* methods. In the first study, the efficacies of pawpaw and

* Corresponding author: John Maina Kagira. Jomo Kenyatta University of Agriculture and Technology, PO Box 62000-00200, Nairobi, Kenya. E-mail: jkagira@yahoo.com, Phone: +254-733986450.

neem products against various stages of *Oesophagostomum* spp were tested under laboratory conditions. The *Oesophagostomum* spp eggs from pigs were exposed to various concentrations of pawpaw, neem products and commercial papain using *in vitro* assays.

Papain and pawpaw latex were the most effective products against *Oesophagostomum* spp, the most lethal effect being on egg hatching with an ED50 ranging between 5 and 59 μg/ml. The adult worms' ED50 was 12.5μg/ml for papain and 25μg/ml for pawpaw latex. In adult worms, the paw paw latex caused the cuticle to disintegrate leading to exposure of internal organs. 100% mortality was observed in adult worms exposed to neem oil concentrations of 25% or higher. The *in vitro* study showed that pawpaw and neem extracts have significant anthelmintics potential. In the second *in vivo* study, the efficacies of pawpaw and neem products were investigated in pigs. Thirty (30) pigs with natural infection of *Oesophagostomum* spp were treated orally with pawpaw latex (1g/Kg), pawpaw seeds powder (1g/Kg), papain (0.3g/Kg), neem oil (0.2ml/Kg) and levamisole (7.5mg/kg) and monitored for egg counts for 56 days post treatment (dpt). Six pigs were also kept as untreated controls. Fecal samples were collected weekly from the pigs and analysed for eggs per gram (EPG) using the McMaster method. Other parameters which were monitored included clinical signs, packed cell volume (PCV) of collected blood and weight changes. The study showed a decline in EPG counts of pigs treated with all the products, with the percentage reductions in EPG at 56dpt in the levamisole, latex, neem, papain, powder treated pigs at 84.6%, 57.1%, 56%, 43.2%, 27.1%, respectively. A rise in mean EPGs (47% at 56 dpt) was observed in the untreated control groups. Significant differences ($p<0.05$) were observed between mean EPGs in the following groups: untreated controls and latex, levamisole and neem groups. There were no clinical signs observed in the treated pigs and the weight gain ranged from 111g to 145g/pig/day, but the weight differences amongst the various groups were not ($p>0.05$) significant. There was an increase in PCV in pigs from all the treatment groups which was higher than that of the untreated control group. It is concluded that, pawpaw products and neem oil used at the current dosages were safe and significant effect against *Oesophagostomum* spp infection in pigs. Further studies on the pawpaw and neem oil products including dosage formulation and effectiveness of the products in integrated control programmes for pig parasites are recommended.

Keywords: *In vitro*, *In vivo*, ED50, *Oesophagostomum* spp, pigs, neem oil, pawpaw latex, seeds, EPG, Kenya

Introduction

Pigs in developing countries are produced under a variety of production systems ranging from intensive commercial pig farms to free-range traditional systems. The farming is faced with several constraints, chief among them being parasitic diseases (Kagira et al., 2011, (Nissen et al., 2011). The most prevalent nematode parasite is *Oesophagostomum* spp. with prevalences of up to 84% being reported in free range production systems (Kagira et al., 2001, Kagira et al., 2001). The parasitic diseases often lead to direct and indirect losses to the resource poor farmers in developing countries, and this warrants development of control strategies. The control of pig nematodes relies almost exclusively on multiple and regular dosing with anthelmintics (Roepstorff and Nansen, 1994; Kagira et al., 2003). However, the use of anthelmintics has several constraints including consumer concerns and development of drug resistance (Conder and Campbell, 1995; Kagira et al., 2003). Thus, in recent years, livestock farmers are encouraged to adopt alternative or novel nematode control methods, plant-based anthelmintics being chief amongst them. The use of ethno-veterinary plant preparations has been documented in different parts of the world (reviewed by Githiori et al., 2006). The importance of ethnoveterinary products in control of pig parasites has not been evaluated in Kenya. A recent study documented that free range pig farmers in the country, used products such as pawpaw seeds to control nematode parasites (Kagira et al., 2009). Pawpaw products, notably, latex has effects against *Heligmosomoides bakeri*, *Aspiculuris tetraptera* and *Hymenolepis nana* infections in mice (Satrija et al., 1994; Stepek et al., 2007). Similarly, plant based latex was observed to have significant effects on gastrointestinal nematodes of humans, *A. suum* in pigs and *Haemonchus controtus* sheep (Hansson et al. 1986; Satrija et al., 1995; Buttle et al., 2011). The efficacy of pawpaw latex against pig nematodes, other than *A. suum*, has however not been tested. Neem (*Azadirachta indica*) products have also been tested against gastrointestinal nematodes of livestock, although they have given inconsistent results (Mitchell et al., 1997, Hordegen et al., 2003, Githiori, 2004, Chandrawathani et al. 2006) which require further evaluation. Previous studies in Kenya have shown that pawpaw products and neem products are commonly used by farmers in control of parasites of domestic animals (Okitoi et al., 2007; Kagira et al., 2009). However, their efficacies against major nematodes of pigs have not been proved in control trials.

The objectives of the current study were:

1 To evaluate the *in vitro* efficacy of pawpaw and neem products against various stages of *Oesophagostomum* spp.
2 To determine the effect of pawpaw latex on the adult *Oesophagostomum* spp was examined at microscopical level.
3 To evaluate the efficacy of pawpaw and neem products in the control of *Oesophagostomum* spp infections of pigs reared under free-range system of production.

Materials and Methods

Products and Their Preparation

The pawpaw latex and seeds were obtained from pawpaw plants (*Carica papaya*) from a farm in Busia District, Kenya. Pawpaw latex was collected as described by Sartrija et al., (1994). A V-shaped incision was made on unripe pawpaw fruits and the latex was collected on the ventral aspect of the incision into universal plastic bottles, weighed, and stored at 4°C until use. Pawpaw seeds were obtained from ripe pawpaw fruits, dried and ground into powder using a grinding machine. The powder was then put into universal bottles and stored at 4°C until use. Neem oil was obtained from a local company (Biolinet-Kenya Ltd, Nairobi, Kenya). The oil was prepared from neem seeds by cold-pressing whole seeds using a vegetable oil expeller. The oil was kept at 4°C before use. Commercially available papain (Cysteine protease, Sigma Ltd, US) was also used. Levamisole (Levamisole HCl, Sigma Ltd, US; Wormicid®, Cosmos Ltd, Kenya) was used as positive control. Before the *in vitro* assays were perfomed the pawpaw seed powder, aqueous extract of seed powder and also latex were dissolved in distilled water to form stock solutions having concentration of 30 mg/ml. Papain and Levamisole were dissolved in distilled water to make a solution of 10mg/ml and 0.5mg/ml, respectively. The effects of various herbal products on *Oesophagostomum* spp was tested using the egg hatch assay, larval mortality assay, larval development assay and adult mortality assay. However, neem oil was only tested for its efficacy against the larvae and adult worms.

In Vitro Study

Faecal Collection and Egg Extraction

Faecal samples were collected from the rectum of naturally infected pigs slaughtered at the Ndumbo-ine slaughter house in Nairobi, Kenya.

Oesopha-gostomum spp eggs were extracted using the method described previously by Hurbert and Kuberof (1992). The cleaned eggs were then collected in a test tube and concentration of the eggs adjusted to 50 eggs per 50μl of distilled water, ready for use in the experiment.

Egg Hatch Assay (EHA)

The Egg Hatch Assay (EHA) was conducted as described by Hurbert and Kuberof (1992) and modified by Maingi et al. (1998) and Thoithi et al. (2002). Serial dilutions of pawpaw aqueous extract, powder, latex were carried out in 96 well plates to give dilutions ranging from 30,000 μg/ml to 15μg/ml of the extracts. Serial dilutions of papain in 96 well plates contained dilutions ranging from 30,000 μg/ml to 4.9 μg/ml.

Serial dilutions of levamisole contained dilutions ranging from 500 μg/ml to 0.244 μg/ml. Control tubes containing distilled water were included in the set-up. 50μl of *Oesophagostomum* spp eggs solution were added into each well and incubated at 27°C for 48hrs.

The number of eggs which had not hatched and number of hatched larvae were counted using the inverted microscope and percent hatching calculated.

Larval Mortality Assay (LMA)

The assay was set-up as described by Thoithi et al. (2002). The initial aspects were undertaken as described for EHA. After determination of the EHA, the plates were incubated for a further 48hrs. The number of live and dead larvae was determined using the inverted microscope and percent death calculated.

Larval Development Assay (LDA)

The LDA was conducted as described by Hurbert and Kuberof (1992) and modified by Maingi et al., (1998). The assay was initially set-up as described for the EHA. The plates were then incubated for 7 days at 27°C. Then, 10 μl of Lugols iodine was added to each well and the number of eggs and larvae that developed to L_3 in each well counted using a dissecting microscope.

Adult Worm Mortality Assay (AWMA)

Adult *Oesophagostomum* spp were collected from the large intestine of naturally infected pigs slaughtered at the Ndumbo-ine slaughter-slab, Nairobi, Kenya. Only worms from pigs without previous anthelmintic treatments were collected. The collected worms were then washed and kept in phosphate buffered saline.

The AWMA was undertaken as described by Houzangbe-Adote et al. (2005). Briefly, the adult worms were placed in petri dishes filled with 4ml of the test products. The pawpaw aqueous extract and powder were prepared in concentrations ranging from 30mg/ml to 1.75mg/ml, while the pawpaw latex and papain preparations ranged from 10mg/ml to 0.125mg/ml. Serial dilutions of Levamisole HCl acted as positive control. After 24 hours the number of motile (alive) and immotile (dead) worms was counted under the dissecting microscope and percentage of dead worms calculated. Morphological changes on the worm were also noted.

Electron Microscopy on Oesophagostomum Spp Exposed to Pawpaw Latex

The electron microscopy work was undertaken as described by Beugnet et al., (1996) with some few modifications. Twenty (20) adult *Oesophagostomum* spp live worms were obtained and exposed to 10 mg/kg of pawpaw latex for 10 minutes as described the above in the AWMA method. Another 20 adult live *Oesophagostomum* worms were kept under physiological saline for 10 minutes and acted as control. The worms were then removed from the petri dishes and fixed in 2% glutaraldehyde diluted in 0.15 phosphate buffered saline (PBS) at pH 7.2 for 48 hours at 4°C. Post fixation of the worms was then undertaken using a mixture of 4% osmium tetroxide for 2 hours as a secondary fixative.

The worms were then dehydrated in increasing concentrations of ethanol (ethanol 70% for 10 minutes, 95% for 20 minutes, 100% for 20 minutes) and then progressively embedded in 'Epon 812' resin. The polymerization lasted 18 hours at 60°C. Thick sections were made, stained with toluidine blue and examined under light microscope to observe the specific areas to be used for ultrathin sectioning. The blocks were then sectioned from 90 to 100 nm thick using a Reichert ultramicrotome (Reichert Jung, Vienna, Austria). These semi-sections were stained with 4% uranyl acetate in aqueous solution for 20 minutes followed by 0.4% lead citrate for 10 minutes. Observations were performed using a Philips 201C Transmission Electron Microscope (TEM), and changes described.

Data Analysis for In Vitro Study

The results were entered into Ms Excel® (Microsoft, US) worksheets before being imported into StatsView® (SAS Institute Inc, 1995–1998, Cary, NC) statistical software where statistical analysis was undertaken. Descriptive statistics were calculated and presented as tables and graphs.

Data from the assays were transformed by probit transformation against logathrim of the plant product concentration.

The extract concentration required to inhibit 50% (ED_{50}) egg hatching, cause 50% (LD_{50}) larval mortality, and prevent 50% (LD_{50}) larvae from developing to L_3 was calculated after correction was made for natural mortality by probit analysis. Comparisons of the mean percentages of egg hatch inhibition and mortality of adult parasites at different concentrations with the control was performed by one-way ANOVA.

Field (*In Vivo*) Study

Pigs and Study Herds

A total of 30 grower pigs from 26 households in the Esikulu village in Busia District were used in the field trial. The pigs used in the study had not been treated with any anthelmintic in the previous 8 weeks, were of either sex, aged between 3 and 6 months of age.

Experimental Design

This was a randomized, controlled efficacy study. At the start of the experiment, the pigs were screened for nematode infections and shown to be infected with *Oesophagostomum* spp (100%). The treatment groups were randomized based on the *Oesophagostomum* spp EPG counts. The study pigs were ear-tagged, screened for nematode egg counts using the McMaster method (MAFF, 1986).

Pigs with an EPG of more than 500 were then randomly allocated into 6 treatment groups of 5 pigs each as detailed in Table 1. The dosages used in the current study were determined from search in literature (Fajimi et al., 2002, Boeke et al., 2004) and doses used by farmers.

Table 1. Treatment regimens for pigs infected with *Oesophagostomum* spp

Group	Treatment	Dosage
1	Pawpaw powder	1g/kg orally
2	Pawpaw latex	1g/kg orally
3	Papain	0.3g/kg orally
4	Neem oil	0.2ml/kg orally
5	Levamisole	7.5mg/kg orally
6	Distilled water	10 ml/pig

After administration of the herbal doses, the pigs were then screened for nematode egg counts at days 7, 14, 28 and 56 days, using McMaster egg counting technique (MAFF, 1986).

To determine any weight changes during the treatment period, the weight of the pigs during sampling points was determined using heart girth tape measure method (Carlson, 2006). During the administration of the herbal products and sampling days, the pigs in the six groups were examined for clinical signs which can be associated with toxicity (e.g., change in stool consistency, raised hair coat, respiratory distress) of the products. Blood was also collected from the jugular vein and analyzed for packed cell volume using the Haematocrit technique (Murray et al., 1977).

Statistical Analysis for In Vivo Study

The results were entered into Ms Excel® worksheets before being imported into StatsView® statistical software where statistical analysis was undertaken. Descriptive statistics were calculated and presented as tables and graphs. The efficacy of various products was undertaken as described in the WAAVP guidelines outlined by Hennesy et al., (2006). The significance of the differences among treatment groups on the mean EPGs was determined using one way ANOVA.

Results

In Vitro Study

All the products had varied effects on *Oesophagostomum* spp and exhibited a linear dose-response relationship. The effective doses of various products on *Oesophagostomum* spp eggs, larvae and adult worms are shown in

Table 2. In descending order, the most effective products against the eggs (EHA) were levamisole, papain, pawpaw latex, pawpaw seed aqueous extract and pawpaw seed powder. For L_1 mortality (LMA) and larval development (LDA), the most effective products were levamisole, latex and papain, while the least effective products were pawpaw seed aqueous extract and pawpaw seed powder. Papain and pawpaw latex were the most effective products against adult worms.

On examination under the light microscope, the pawpaw latex and papain affected the cuticle of the adult worms leading to erosion of outer cuticle of the worm, weakening and formation of crinkled ridges.

Table 2. Anthelmintic activity (ED_{50}) of various pawpaw plant products against various stages of *Oesophagostomum* spp

Plant product/anthelmintic	ED_{50} (μg/ml) values of different assays			
	EHA	LMA	LDA	AWMA
Pawpaw seed aqueous extract	234	3750	2362	2572
Pawpaw seed powder	554	3050	938	4743
Pawpaw latex	59	117	371	25
Commercial papain	5	31.25	20.8	12.5
Levamisole	0.8	0.5	0.18	ND

Key: EHA=Egg hatch assay, LMA= Larval (L_1) mortality assay, LDA= Larval development assay, AWMA = Adult worm mortality assay, ND = Not done.

In some worms, the cuticle weakened and burst at some points leading to exposure of internal organs and eggs. At high doses of 10 - 30 mg/kg, the latex and papain completely dissolved the worm within a period of 12 hours. At electron microscopy (EM) a similar process was observed to occur within the cuticle structure.

Apart from features described above, at EM the cuticle was also observed to become weak and underwent disintegration and this lead to formation of empty halos within all the layers of cuticle. The hypodermis layer also appeared to become lighter, while in other sections there was separation from both the upper cuticle and lower muscular layers.

For adult worms, the LD_{50} of neem oil was a concentration of 6.25% (24 hrs). 100% mortality was observed in adult worms exposed to neem oil concentrations of 25% or higher. For larvae, the LD_{50} of neem oil was 25%. 100% mortality was achieved when larvae were exposed to neem oil at concentrations of 50% or higher. Neem oil appeared to form oil droplets along the cuticle of the worm, causing disruption of the cuticle. However, the disruption of the cuticle was not as severe as that of the pawpaw latex.

Field (*In Vivo* Study)

The EPG levels in pigs treated with various products are shown in Figure 1. At day 0, there were no significant differences (p=0.68) in the *Oesophagostomum* spp EPGs of the various groups. In all the treated groups, the mean EPGs declined when compared with those at day zero.

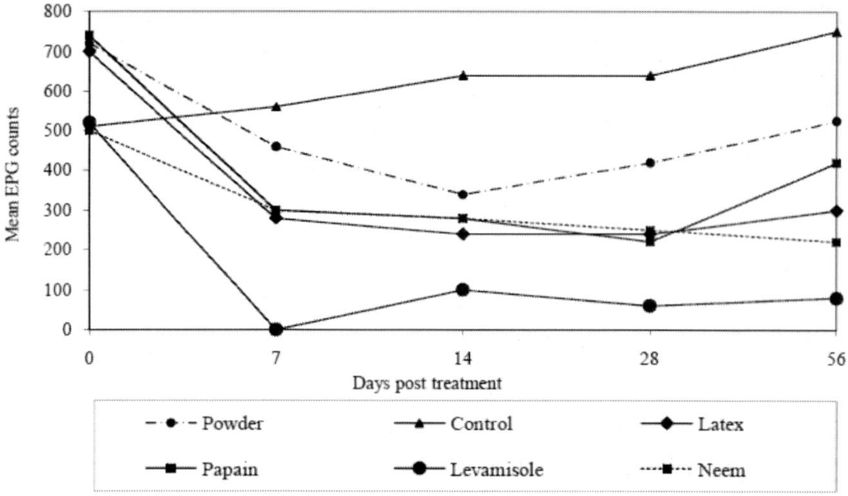

Figure 1. Egg per gram (EPG) counts in pigs treated with various plant products.

Thus, the overall decline in mean EPGs were statistically significant for the groups treated with pawpaw powder (F=5.12, p=0.007), latex (F=3.95, p=0.02), papain (F=2.96, p=0.052), neem oil (F=3.78, p=0.02) and levamisole. However, there was a significant (F=3.04, p=0.048) increase in mean EPG counts in pigs in the untreated control group during the monitoring period. At 56 days post treatment, there were significant differences (p<0.05) between mean EPGs in the control group and those of latex, levamisole and neem oil groups.

Further, there was significant difference (p=0.03) in mean EPGs of the levamisole and powder treated groups at 56 days post treatment.

The percentage reduction in mean EPGs were also analysed across the different treatment groups as shown in Figure 2. The maximum reduction in mean EPGs for the treatment groups included: Levamisole group at day 7 (100%), papain group at day 28 (70.8%), pawpaw latex group at day 14 and 28 (65.7%), pawpaw powder at day 14 (52.8%) and neem oil group at day 28 (50%).

At the end of the study (56 days post treatment), the percentage reductions in mean EPG in the levamisole, latex, neem oil, papain, powder treated groups was 84.6%, 57.1%, 56%, 43.2%, 27.1%, respectively. The increase in mean EPG counts in pigs in the untreated control group was 21.8%, 39.1%, 39.1% and 47% at 7, 14, 28 and 56 days post treatment, respectively.

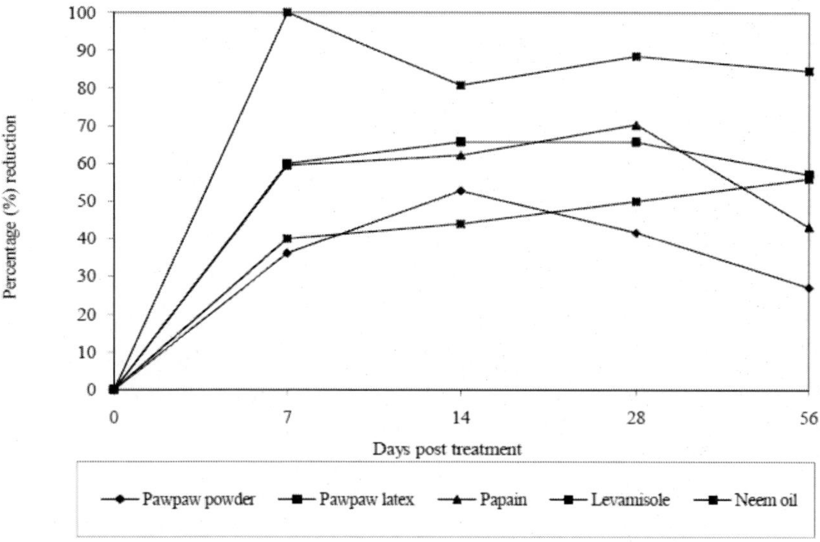

Figure 2. Percentage reduction of egg per gram (EPG) counts in pigs administered various plant products.

The treated pigs did not develop any clinical symptom which could be associated with toxicity. In all the groups, there was an increase in body weights by day 56, where a mean increment of 8.1, 7.7, 6.8, 6.3, and 6.2 Kgs was observed in pigs treated with neem oil, powder, papain, levamisole and latex, respectively.

Thus, the daily weight gain ranged from 145g to 111 g/pig/day. The control group had a mean increment of 5.5 Kgs (98g/pig/day). The increase of weight was significantly ($p<0.05$) related to days post treatment in the neem oil, powder, papain and levamisole treated groups, but not ($p>0.05$) in latex and control groups. However, comparisons of the weight changes in the different groups were not significant ($p>0.05$).

The PCV of all the groups increased with time. In descending order, the highest increment of PCV at 56 days post treatment was observed in pigs treated with levamisole (3.8%), neem oil (3%), papain (2.1%), latex (2%) and lowest increment was in pigs treated with pawpaw powder (1.6%). There was also an increment of PCV in the untreated infected pigs (1%) at 56 days post treatment. The mean PCV was not significantly ($p>0.05$) related to sampling date in all the treatment groups. However, the mean PCV levels at 28 days post treatment in the control group were significantly ($p<0.05$) lower than those in the levamisole and neem groups.

Discussion

In Vitro Study

The plant products used in the current study had *in vitro* effects against a gastro-intestinal nematode *Oesophagostomum* spp. The pawpaw products (latex and papain) significantly affected the 3 key lifecycle stages of *Oesophagostomum* spp, that is eggs, larvae and adult worms, indicating their potential as anthelmintics.

Generally, papain and paw paw latex were the most effective products against *Oesophagostomum* spp, the most lethal effect being on egg hatching and the survival of adult worms. By affecting these two stages of the parasites, the products can affect the normal physiology and anatomy of the adult worms and also affect the viability of eggs excreted by pigs to the environment.

The lethal doses (LD_{50}) were however higher than that of levamisole and those reported for benzimidazoles (Varady et al., 1996).

Papain is an extract from pawpaw latex which has been shown to be efficacious against nematodes such as *Ascaris suum*, *Hemonchus contortus* and several helminths of mice (Satrija et al., 1994, Stepek et al., 2007, Buttle et al., 2011).

The current study reports for the first time the effect of paw paw latex and papain on *Oesophagostomum* spp. The LD_{50} of papain and crude pawpaw latex against motility of the mice nematode *H. bakeri* was reported as 7.5 and 12.5μM (Behnke et al., 2008), values which are lower than those reported in this study. The variation could be related to other factors including amount of active ingredients in the products used as well as host and parasite differences.

On the other hand, the pawpaw seeds and the water extract from seeds had moderate effect on egg hatching and had minimal effects on larval development and adult worms.

This shows that there were some water soluble active principles in the seeds. Alcohol extracts of *C. papaya* seeds were also shown to affect the egg hatching, larval migration and adult worm motility of *H. contortus* and *T. colubriformis* by Houzangbe-Adote et al. (2005). For *H. contortus* and *T. colubriformis*, the percent immobile adult worms at 2500μg/ ml concentration of the pawpaw extract were 100% and 38.1% respectively (Houzangbe-Adote et al., 2005).

In contrast, the current study reported the LD_{50} for aqueous extract and seed powder against adult worms of *Oesophagostomum* spp as 2,572μg/ml and 4,743μg/ml, respectively.

The pawpaw latex and papain appeared to have similar effects on the adult worms, mainly affecting the cuticle of the adult worms. The observed lesions included loss of normal architecture of the cuticle, formation of crinkled ridges, bursting and erosion of the cervical vesicle. At higher concentrations (>15mg/ml), the products caused the worms to disintegrate. The cuticle mainly consists of collagen-like proteins cross-linked by disulphide bonds (Behnke et al., 2008) and it is possible that the proteinases (in pawpaw latex) could be targeting these bonds, resulting in weakening of the cuticle at mainly the basal and medial layers.

The role of protease is also critical during molting, where an exsheathment protease is responsible for dissolution of hypordermis and basal layers of cuticle (Wharton, 1991). During the current study, it was observed that on exposure to the papain and pawpaw latex, the outermost layer of the worms' cuticle crinkled and the ridges lost their rigidity.

Neem oil was effective against the larvae and adult worms at concentrations above 6.25%. The effect of neem oil on animal nematodes has not been earlier reported in published literature. Other products of neem plants have been shown to have some efficacy against a number of livestock nematodes (Ahmed, 1994, Chandrawathani et al., 2006). In sheep, neem kernel powder was shown to cause a decrease in nematode eggs and an increase in body weight (Ahmed, 1994).

Chandrawathani et al. (2006) reported that *ad libitum* feeding of fresh neem leaves produced 82% reduction in worm eggs, while a study by Githiori (2004) did not reveal any significant reduction by neem extracts on helminth infections in mice and sheep. The higher level of Azidachtrin A concentration, an active molecule against parasites, in neem oil (25mg/100g) compared to only 0.59mg/100g (Sindaram, 1996) in leaves could partly explain the significant effect reported in this study.

In the current study, the neem oil appeared to form droplets along the cuticle lining, thereby disrupting the normal structure of the cuticle. It has been reported that apart from effects of azadirachtin, clarified hydrophobic extracts of neem oil can possibly cause death of parasites through either disruption of the outer membrane/cuticles and/or interference with respiration (Mitchell et al., 1997). Further studies on the effect of higher doses of neem oil on pig nematodes should be evaluated.

In conclusion, this study has demonstrated that pawpaw and neem oil products have significant *in vitro* efficacy against *Oesophagostomum* spp. The effects of pawpaw latex on *Oesophagostomum* spp was be attributed to destruction of the parasite's cuticle.

Further studies on the pawpaw and neem oil products should be carried out in pigs to determine the effectiveness of these products in control of *Oesophagostomum* spp and other nematodes of pigs.

In Vivo Study

In the field (*in vivo*) study, the pawpaw and neem products were tested against *Oesophagostomum* spp, a common nematode in pigs.

All the administered products had varied effects on the fecal egg counts. Levamisole, the positive control drug, caused 100% reduction in worm counts 7 days post treatment and this showed the drug is highly effective against pig nematodes. Levamisole is the most common conventional drug used by the pig farmers in Kenya, possibly because it is cheap and readily available (Kagira et al., 2009). The less than 90% efficacy of levamisole at days 14 and 28 implies either an occurrence of anthelmintic resistance or under strength drug, which should be further investigated. The occurrence of *Oesophagostomum* spp resistant to levamisole and the use of substandard anthelmintics have been reported to occur in Kenya (Kagira et al., 2003).

The *in vivo* studies showed that papain and pawpaw latex were the most effective pawpaw products, causing an EPG reduction of 70.3% and 65.7%, respectively at day 28 post treatment. It is important to note that pigs infected with *Oesophagostomum* spp do not develop immunity against this worm, and thus reduction of worm burden due to development of immunity was not suspected. In the current study, the latex and papain were administered at 1 mg/kg and thus it is possible that higher doses will cause a higher reduction in worm burdens. However, it should be noted that pawpaw latex might not affect developmental stages of the *Oesophagostomum* spp, which are located within the mucosa. The larval stages in the mucosa may be responsible for increase in EPG at 56 days post treatment and thus the need for multiple treatments. Similarly, mucosal stages of *H. bakeri* and *T. muris* were not affected by pawpaw latex (Behnke et al., 2008). This may be a useful property; where treatment with latex will be stage-specific damaging only the adult worms and leaving out the developmental stages which can repopulate the gut subsequently.

As suggested by van Wyk, (2001), this may slow any development of anthelmintic resistance, although this would mean that treatments would have to be repeated frequently where exposure to infective stages is high.

Alternatively, the animals can be regularly fed supplements with raw pawpaws. Pawpaw seed powder was least in causing the fecal egg count reduction (36.1% at day 7, 52.8% at day 14, 41.7% at day 28 and 27.1% at day 56). It is important to note that a substantial number of farmers in Busia District, Kenya used pawpaw seed to deworm their pigs (Kagira et al., 2009). The farmers had indicated that they used a handful of seeds which they fed to their pigs. Since a handful will vary from individual to individual administering the seeds, the variation of amount given by farmers could be wide. However, quantitatively, the amount of seeds given in this study (>30g/pig) appeared far above that given by farmers, and thus the efficacies claimed by farmers might not be justifiable.

Reports of the effect of pawpaw seeds on gastrointestinal nematodes are scarce. Fajimi et al., (2002) reported that dried pawpaw seeds administered at 50mg/kg, twice a week for 6 weeks (total dose =600mg/kg) to sheep, caused the EPGs of *Oesophagostomum* spp, *Trichuris*, and *Trichostrongylus* spp to reduce by 87%, 95% and 93%, respectively. Pawpaw seeds also caused 80% reduction in fecal egg counts in sheep (Hounzangbe-Adotte et al., 2001). The mode of administration, quality of seeds used, geographical differences of cultivated pawpaw, host and parasite differences could have influenced the variation between these studies. Future experiments should evaluate the higher doses of pawpaw seeds as well their extracts (e.g., alcohol) to determine their efficacies against the nematodes of pigs.

At the doses used in the field study, neem oil had moderate efficacy against the *Oesophagostomum* spp. The effect of neem oil on animal nematodes has not been earlier reported in published literature. Other products of neem plants have been shown to have some efficacy against a number of livestock nematodes (Ahmed, 1994; Chandrawathani et al., 2006). In sheep, neem kernel powder was shown to cause a decrease in nematode eggs and an increase in body weight (Ahmed, 1994). Chandrawathani et al., (2006) reported that *ad libitum* feeding of fresh neem leaves produced 82% reduction in worm eggs, while a study by Githiori (2004) did not reveal any significant reduction by neem extracts on helminth infections in mice and sheep. The higher level of Azidachtrin A concentration in neem oil (~25mg/100g) compared to only ~0.59/100g (Sindaram, 1996) in leaves could partly explain the moderate effects observed in the current study. In the current study, the neem oil appeared to form droplets along the cuticle lining, thereby disrupting the normal structure of the cuticle. It has been reported that apart from effects of azadirachtin, clarified hydrophobic extracts of neem oil can possibly cause death of parasites through disruption of the outer membrane/cuticles and/or interference with respiration. Further studies on the effect of higher doses of neem oil on pig nematodes should be evaluated.

In spite of the decline in EPG counts in the treated groups, the weight changes in the different groups were not significantly different from that of controls, although the mean weight in the latter group was the lowest. It is possible that the period of monitoring was not long enough to allow the weight gain differences to be significant. Further, the weight gains of all the groups were quite low considering the pigs used were growers. The daily weight gain (DWG) ranging between 111-145g /day was low compared to other studies where pig growers are expected to have DWG of more than 300g/day (Nguyen et al., 1997). This could be explained by the fact that pigs in our study were crossbreeds with poor productive potential and were mainly grazers which were not fed substantial supplements. In Vietnam, the mean daily live weight gain of pigs under the traditional feeding system was observed to be low (202-230 g/day) but was significantly increased to between 363-and 366 g/day by giving the protein supplement (Nguyen et al., 1997).

The pigs administered with the various plant products did not manifest any clinical sign that could be associated with toxicity. Others studies have shown that high doses of pawpaw latex (8mg/kg) produce diarrhea and constipation in pigs (Satrija et al., 1994) and mice (Satrija et al., 1995). Purified enzymes from pawpaw have also been observed to have low toxicity to humans, thus chymopapain is a licensed drug for treatment of inter-vertebral disc disease in human beings, while proteases have been used as meat tenderizers (Behnke et al., 2008).

In conclusion, the current study showed that pawpaw products and neem oil were efficacious against *Oesophagostomum* spp, a common nematode which have deleterious effects on health and production of pigs. The effects were observed in both laboratory assays and field trials. In view of the fact that conventional anthelmintics are expensive and unaffordable to resource poor small scale farmers, these novel products should be integrated in the control measures of helminth parasites in pigs.

Acknowledgments

The study was funded by the Lake Victoria Research Initiative (VICRES) and Kenya Agricultural Productivity Program (KAPP). The authors are grateful to the assistance provided by Mr. Boniface Ouma in the collection of the pawpaw seeds and latex.

Other forms of assistance were contributed by Administrative Officers (providing logistics), technical staff of KARI-TRC (animal handling and collection of samples) and farmers who allowed their pigs to be used in the current study.

References

Ahmed, M. (1994). Nematicidal potential of the Neem tree *Azadirachta indica* (A. Juss). *Integrated Pest Management Reviews* 5, 57-66.

Behnke, J. M., Buttle, D. J., Stepek, G., Lowe, A., and Duce, I. R. (2008). Developing novel anthelmintics from plant cysteine proteinases. *Parasite and Vectors* 1, 29-31.

Boeke, S. J., Boersma, M. G., Alink, G. M., Loon, J. J. A., Huis, A., Dicke, M., and Rietjens, M. C. M. (2004): Safety evaluation of neem (*Azadirachta indica*) derived pesticides. *Journal of Ethnopharmacology*, 94, 25-41.

Beugnet, F., Kerboeuf, D., Nicolle, J. C., and Soubieux, D., (1996). Use of free living stages to study the effects of thiabendazole, levamisole, pyrantel and ivermectin on the fine structure of *Haemonchus contortus* and *Heligmosomoides polygyrus*. *Veterinary Parasitology*, 63, 83-94.

Buttle, D. J., Behnke, J. M., Bartley, Y., Elsheikha, H. M., Bartley, D. J., Garnett, M. C., Donnan, A. A., Jackson, F., Lowe, A., and Duce, I. R.,

(2011). Oral dosing with pawpaw latex is an effective anthelmintic treatment for sheep infected with *Haemonchus contortus. Parasite and Vectors* 15; 36 -37.

Carlson, M. (2006). Pig's weight from measurements. University of Missouri Extension manual. University of Missouri. http://extension.missouri.edu/p/G2520.

Chandrawathani, P., Chang, K. W., Nurulaini, L., Waller, P. J., and Vincent, N. (2006). Daily feeding of fresh Neem leaves for worm control in sheep. *Tropical Biomedicine* 23, 23-30.

Conder, G. A. and Campbell, W. C. (1995). Chemotherapy of nematode infections of veterinary importance with special reference to drug resistance. *Advances in Parasitology*, 35, 1-84.

Fajimi, A. K., Taiwo, A. A., Ayodeji, I. O., Adebowale, E. A., and Ogundola, F. I. (2002). Therapeutic trials on gastrointestinal helminth parasite of goats using pawpaw seeds as a drench. Proceedings of the international conference on sustainable crop and livestock production. *Livestock production for improved livelihoods and natural resources management.* International Livestock Research Institute (ILRI) Nov. 9–23, 2001.

Githiori, J. B. (2004): Evaluation of anthelmintic properties of ethnoveterinary plant preparations used as livestock dewormers by pastoralists and small holder farmers in Kenya. *PhD Thesis. Swedish University of Agricultural Sciences,* Uppsala, Sweden.

Githiori, J. B., Athanasiadou, S. and Thamsborg, S. M. (2006). Use of plants in novel approaches for control of gastrointestinal helminths in livestock with emphasis on small ruminants. *Veterinary Parasitology*, 139, 308-320.

Hansson, A., Veliz, G., Naquira, C., Amren, M., Arroyo, M., and Arevalo, G., (1986). Preclinical and clinical studies with latex from *Ficus glabrata* HBK, a traditional intestinal anthelminthic in the Amazonian area. *Journal of Ethnopharmacology,* 17, 105-138.

Hennesy, D. R., Bauer, C., Boray, J. C., Conder, G. A., Daugschies, A., Johansen, M. V., Maddox-Hyttel, C., and Roepstorff, A., (2006). WAAVP: Second edition of guidelines for evaluating the efficacy of anthelmintics in swine. *Veterinary Parasitology*, 141, 138-149.

Hordegen, P., Hertzberg, H., Heilman, J., Langhans, W., and Maurer, V., (2003). The anthelmintic efficacy of five plant products against gastro-intestinal trichostrongylids in artificially infected lambs. *Veterinary Parasitology*, 117, 51-60.

Hounzangbe-Adote, M. S., Paolini, V., Fouraste, I., Moutairou, K., and Hoste, H., (2005). *In vitro* effects of four tropical plants on three life-cycle stages of the parasitic nematode, *Haemonchus contortus. Research in Veterinary Science*, 78, 155-60.

Hounzangbe-Adote, M. S., Zinsou, E., Affognon, K. J., Koutinhouin, B., Adamou, M., and Moutairou, K., (2001). Efficacité antiparasitaire de la poudre de graines de papaye (Carica papaya) sur les strongles gastro-intestinaux des moutons Djallonké au sud du Bénin. *Revue d'elevage et de Medecine Veterinaire des pays Tropicaux*, 54, 225-229.

Hubert, J. and Kerbouef, D., (1992). A microlarval development assay for detection of anthelmintic resistance in sheep nematodes. *Veterinary Record*, 130, 442-446.

Kagira, J. M., Kanyari, P. W. N., Maingi, N., Githigia, S. M., Ng'ang'a, J. C., and Karuga, J. W., (2009). Characteristics of the smallholder free-range pig production system in western Kenya. *Tropical Animal Health and Production*, 42, 865–873.

Kagira, J. M., Githigia, S. M., Maingi, N., Kanyari, P. W., Ng'ang'a, J. C., and Gachohi, J. M., (2011). Risk factors associated with occurrence of nematodes in free-range pigs in Busia district, Kenya. *Tropical Animal Health and Production*, DOI 10.1007/s11250-011-9951-9.

Kagira, J. M., Waruiru, R. M., Munyua, W. K., and Kanyari, P. W. N., (2001). The prevalence of gastrointestinal parasites in commercial pig farms in Thika district, Kenya. *Bulletin of Animal Health and Production in Africa*, 50, 1-8.

Kagira, J. M., Kanyari, P. W. N., Munyua, W. K., and Waruiru, R. M., (2003). The control of parasitic nematodes in commercial piggeries in Kenya as reflected by a questionnaire survey on management practices. *Tropical Animal Health and Production*, 35, 79-84.

Maingi, N., Bjørn, H. and Dangolla, A., (1998). The relationship between faecal egg count reduction and the lethal dose 50% in the egg hatch assay and larval development assay. *Veterinary Parasitology*, 77, 133-145.

MAFF, (1986). Ministry of Agriculture, Fisheries and Food (MAFF). *Manual of Veterinary Parasitological Laboratory Techniques*, 3rd edn., reference book 418. HMSO, London.

Mitchell, M. J., Smith, S. L., Johnson, S., and Morgan, E. D., (1997). Effects of the neem tree compounds azadirachtin, salannin, nimbin, and 6-desacetylnimbin on ecdysone 20-monooxygenase activity. *Archives on Insect Biochemistry and Physiology*, 35, 199-209.

Murray, M., Murray, P. K. and McIntyre, W. I., (1977). An improved parasitological technique for the diagnosis of African trypanosomiasis.

Transaction Royal Society of Tropical Medicine and Hygiene, 71, 325-326.

Nissen, S., Poulsen, I. H., Nejsum, P., Olsen, A., Roepstorff, A., Rubaire-Akiiki, C., Thamsborg, S. M., (2011). Prevalence of gastrointestinal nematodes in growing pigs in Kabale District in Uganda. *Tropical Animal Health and Production,* 43, 567–572.

Nguyen T. L., Ogle B. and Preston T. R., (1997). Protein supplementation of traditional diets for crossbred pigs under village conditions in Central Vietnam. *Livestock Research for Rural Development* 9: http://www.cipav.org.co/lrrd/lrrd9/2/loc921.html.

Okitoi, L. O., Ondwasy, H. O., Siamba D. N., and Nkurumah D., 2007. Traditional herbal preparations for indigenous poultry health management in Western Kenya. *Livestock Research for Rural Development* 19: http://www.cipav.org.co/lrrd/lrrd19/5/okit19072.htm.

Roepstorff, A. and Nansen, P., (1994). Epidemiology and control of helminth infection in pigs under intensive and non-intensive production systems. *Veterinary Parasitology*, 54, 69-85.

Satrija, F., Nansen, P., Bjørn, H., Murtini, S., and He, S. (1994). Effect papaya latex (*Carica papaya*) against *Ascaris suum* in naturally infected pigs. *Journal of Helminthology*, 68, 343-346.

Satrija, F., P. Nansen, S. Murtini and He, S., (1995). Anthelmintic activity of papaya latex against patent *Heligmosomoides polygyrus* infections in mice. *Journal of Ethnopharmacology*, 48, 161-164.

Sindaram, K. M. S., (1996). Azidachtrin biopesticide: a review of studies conducted on its analystical chemistry, environment behaviour and biological effects. *Journal of Enviromental Science and Health*, 13, 913-948.

Stepek, G., Lowe, A. E., Buttle, D. J., Duce, I. R., and Behnke, J. M., (2007). The anthelmintic efficacy of plant-derived cysteine proteinases against the rodent gastrointestinal nematode, *Heligmosomoides polygyrus, in vivo. Parasitology*, 134, 1409-1419.

Thoithi, G. N., Maingi, N., Karume, D., Gathumbi, P. K., Mwangi, J. W., and Kibwage, I. O., (2002). Anthelmintic and other pharmacological activities of the root bark extracts of *Albizia anthelmintica* Brongn. East and Central Africa. *Journal of Pharmaceutical Sciences*, 5, 60-66.

Varady, M., Bjorn, H. and Nansen, P., (1996). *In-vitro* characterisation of anthelmintic susceptibility of field isolates of the pig nodular worm *Oesophagostomum* spp. susceptible or resistant to various anthelmintics. *International Journal for Parasitology*, 26, 733-740.

Van Wyk, J. A., (2001). Refugia—overlooked as perhaps the most potent factor concerning the development of anthelmintic resistance. *Onderstepoort Journal Veterinary Research*, 68, 55–67.

Wharton, D. A., (1991). Ultrastructural changes associated with exsheathment of infective juveniles of *Caenorhabditis elegans*. *Journal of Microscopy*, 164, 187-188.

Index

A

B

C

D

E

F

G

H

I

J

N

O

P

Q

R

S

T